Basic Counseling Skills for Higher Education Professionals

NASPA.
Student Affairs Administrators
in Higher Education

REBEKAH F. SCHULZE AND MAUREEN C. KENNY

Basic Counseling Skills for Higher Education Professionals

Identifying and Addressing Mental Health Concerns

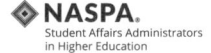

Student Affairs Administrators
in Higher Education

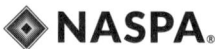
Student Affairs Administrators
in Higher Education

Copyright © 2023 by the National Association of Student Personnel Administrators (NASPA), Inc. All rights reserved.

Published by
NASPA–Student Affairs Administrators in Higher Education
111 K Street, NE
10th Floor
Washington, DC 20002
www.naspa.org

No part of this publication may be reproduced, stored in a retrieval system, or transmitted in any form or by any means, now known or hereafter invented, including electronic, mechanical, photocopying, recording, scanning, information storage and retrieval, or otherwise, except as permitted under Section 107 of the 1976 United States Copyright Act, without the prior written permission of the Publisher.

Additional copies may be purchased by contacting the NASPA publications department at 202-265-7500 or visiting http://bookstore.naspa.org.

NASPA does not discriminate on the basis of race; color; national origin; religion; sex; age; gender identity or expression; affectional or sexual orientation; veteran status; disability; marital status; personal appearance; family responsibilities; genetic information; educational status; political affiliation; place of residence or business; source of income; caste; matriculation; credit information; status as a survivor or family member of a survivor of domestic violence, a sexual offense, or stalking; reproductive health decision making; or any other basis protected by law in any of its policies, programs, publications, and services. NASPA prohibits discrimination and harassment at any time, including during its events or within publications and online learning communities.

Library of Congress Cataloging-in-Publication Data

Names: Schulze, Rebekah F., author. | Kenny, Maureen C., 1967- author.
Title: Basic counseling skills for higher education professionals : identifying and addressing mental health concerns / Rebekah F. Schulze and Maureen C. Kenny.
Description: Washington, DC : NASPA–Student Affairs Administrators in Higher Education, [2023] | Includes bibliographical references and index.
Identifiers: ISBN: 978-1948213387 (paperback) | 978-1948213394 (ebook)
Subjects: LCSH: Counseling in higher education. | College students—Mental health. | College administrators—Training of.
Classification: LCC: LB2343 .S38 2023 | DDC: 378.194—dc23

Printed and bound in the United States of America

FIRST EDITION

Contents

1. Introduction 1

2. Basic Counseling Skills 7

3. Setting Boundaries and Understanding Confidentiality 25

4. Stages of Change and Making Referrals 33

5. Self-Care 43

6. Cultural and Diversity Awareness 59

7. Anxiety and Stress 71

8. Depression and Suicide 87

9. Eating Disorders 103

10. Sexual Assault and Victimization 123

11. Interpersonal Violence 143

12. Substance Abuse 159

13. Grief and Loss 181

14. Moving Forward 193

Appendix: Mental Health Resources 197

The Authors 213

Index 215

CHAPTER 1

Introduction

College is an exciting time, one that is often described as "the best 4 years of your life." That may be true. For many, it can be a time of transition, growth, and challenge; for others, it is also a time of pressure and confusion. Some enter college with preexisting mental health issues and a history of struggle, including problems with drugs and alcohol and past victimization. If these issues are unresolved, the stress of college life can often heighten them.

In a 2019 American Council on Education study, college presidents cited mental health as their number one concern for their students—ranked even higher than the financial stability of their own institutions (Chessman & Taylor, 2019). The American College Health Association (2022) National College Health Assessment further demonstrated the need for increased attention to the mental well-being of today's college students. More than 70,000 college students across the nation responded, and the statistics are concerning. Almost 6% said they had attempted suicide in the last 12 months. Another 16% said they had planned an attempt, and another 27%

had thought about it. That's almost half of respondents thinking, planning, or attempting suicide. More than 80% claimed that their stress levels were either moderate or high. Almost all students responded that in the past 12 months, they felt nervous some, most, or all of the time; yet, of these respondents, only 28% had received any sort of counseling.

These statistics, while alarming, are not surprising. When students find themselves in a crisis, they will likely turn to a peer, trusted faculty member, or staff member first. These interactions are often unhelpful, leaving students feeling further isolated, confused, and still in need of help. Drum et al. (2009) found that among students with serious suicidal ideation and attempts, 46% said they never talked to anyone else about these issues, and of those students who did talk to someone else, 67% of the time it was a peer—most often a close friend or roommate. Of those who talked about their struggles with others, only 52% found it helpful and only 58% were advised to seek professional help. This means that most students have no real professional help for their often very serious mental health issues.

As the number of students in crisis continues to rise, higher education professionals continue to be called upon to do more. Their roles have gone far beyond that of administrator alone. After the tragic shootings at Virginia Tech in 2007, a clear reevaluation of how higher education administrators responded to students in distress took place. New focus was placed on policies, procedures, and protocols (Jablonski et al., 2008). As the need to assist students continues to rise, the best ways to help them are still being explored. Pressure, however, continues to be placed on higher education professionals to intervene and be ready when approached. The statistics from the 2021 ACHA survey attest that higher education professionals often find themselves not only managing their own administrative duties but also helping students with their stress and mental health needs (Becker & Drum, 2015). This book aims to give higher education professionals the knowledge and skills necessary to intervene in ways that are effective and that can contribute to positive outcomes for students.

Training and Preparation

A good way to start reading this book is with the understanding that everyone struggles. We all have what we call our "stuff"—whatever it is that bothers us, causes us to worry, makes us feel stress, or gives us anxiety. The specific "stuff" may be different for every person, but we all have it, this *universality of struggle*. This is not an "us versus them" situation where those of us reading this book are the mentally healthy ones looking to help those who are not. Again: We all have our "stuff." Recognizing and accepting this fact helps to destigmatize mental health issues. When we verbalize our own "stuff," we are letting others know they are not alone in their struggles. Although such articulation has improved in recent years, with celebrities, musicians, and athletes willingly coming forward to discuss their personal struggles with mental health issues, more work remains to be done to reduce the stigma associated with mental health.

The Backpack Metaphor

Often, we think that getting rid of our "stuff" will make everything better. But that is not usually the case—usually, it only gets worse. Let's explore this idea through a backpack metaphor, developed by Charlie Morse (personal communication, August 30, 2007), the director of the Student Development Counseling Center at Worcester Polytechnic Institute. When we take our backpack and put all our stuff in it, we will most likely carry it on our back. That's how it's designed, right? Eventually, though, it will start to get heavy. We could hand it to someone else, and they might carry it for a while, but eventually they are just going to give it back. They'll remind us that it is our stuff, and we need to figure out how to carry it in a way that is healthy. After all, we need this backpack for a long time. So, maybe we put the backpack down and walk away from it. That might work, but most likely someone is going to find it and return it anyhow. Once again, we will need to figure out how to deal with this weight. So, what's the best way to carry this heavy backpack? In front. Where we can see it, face it, protect it, and accept it. We may also want to get rid of some of the things inside—maybe coping skills or habits that are not working for us anymore. This book is designed to help higher education professionals work with students to "manage their stuff," to help students find ways to put that backpack in front of them, where it become less heavy and easier to manage.

Higher education professionals, however, are not always prepared to help students "carry their backpacks." They might have had a class in their graduate program or attended a professional development training or two. Perhaps they have enrolled in courses within the clinical counseling programs at their institutions, but those courses tend to be geared more toward students planning to enter clinical practice. Sometimes, higher education students are prevented from enrolling in these classes because seats are needed for students majoring in those degrees. Some higher education curriculums may not address mental health issues at all. More instruction is needed to prepare higher education professionals for assisting with students' mental health issues.

How to Help

Counseling centers often take the lead on campuses in providing leadership for mental health education and outreach activities. But to be effective, they must involve the entire campus community. Such efforts will help build trust among stakeholders and encourage conversations about mental health issues, which can reduce mental health stigma (Morse & Schulze, 2013). Higher education professionals can often find themselves in situations where they feel ill-prepared to respond to students who are struggling. They might feel it is not their place to discuss personal matters with their students, or they feel they lack the knowledge and expertise necessary to be helpful. They want the confidence to have these important conversations but instead shy away from approaching students about whom they are concerned. In this book, we want to give higher education professionals enough information to understand common mental health issues they might encounter on campus—but not so much information to overwhelm them. Higher education professionals need not be experts in mental health disorders and their etiologies; they simply need to understand basic signs and symptoms and know how to listen and show empathy. They need to know when it is time for more trained professionals to step in and help. It is the responsibility of mental health counselors to go deeper in diagnoses and treatments. The chapters in this book will provide a basic knowledge of what is needed to feel prepared to address and respond to students who are struggling.

References

American College Health Association. (2022). *American College Health Association–National College Health Assessment III: Reference group executive summary spring 2022.* https://www.acha.org/documents/ncha/NCHA-III_SPRING_2022_REFERENCE_GROUP_EXECUTIVE_ SUMMARY.pdf

Becker, M. S., & Drum, D. J. (2015). The influence of suicide prevention gatekeeper training on resident assistants' mental health. *Journal of Student Affairs Research and Practice, 52*(1), 76–88. https://doi.org/10.1080/19496591.2015.996055

Chessman, H., & Taylor, M. (2019, August 12). College student mental health and well-being: A survey of presidents. *Higher Education Today.* https://www.higheredtoday.org/2019/08/12/college-student-mental-health-well-survey-college-presidents

Drum, D. J., Brownson, C., Denmark, A. B., & Smith, S. E. (2009). New data on the nature of suicidal crises in college students: Shifting the paradigm. *Professional Psychology: Research and Practice, 40*(3), 213–222. https://doi.org/10.1037/a0014465

Jablonski, M., McClellan, G., & Zdziarski, E. (2008). *In search of safer communities: Emerging practices for student affairs in addressing campus violence* (New Directions for Student Services). Jossey-Bass.

Morse, C., & Schulze, R. (2013). Enhancing the network of peer support on college campuses. *Journal of College Student Psychotherapy, 27*(3), 212–225. https://doi.org/10.1080/87566225.2013.798222

CHAPTER 2

Basic Counseling Skills

This chapter will present an overview of the basic counseling skills higher education professionals need to be successful in their roles. The primary listening skills, including attending, summarizing, and reflecting feeling and content, will be reviewed, drawing on the work of Alan Ivey. Readers will learn how to listen to a student and elicit necessary information. Basic listening skills are critical to forming good working relationships with others and can help set the stage for future interactions. The chapter will explore the role of empathic helping and listening, while taking care not to impose one's own values.

Counseling in Higher Education

Even if you are not trained to be a counselor, possessing some basic counseling skills will assist you in your work with students. *Counseling* is defined as "a professional relationship that empowers diverse individuals, families and groups to accomplish mental health, wellness, education and career goals. It involves the application of cognitive, affective, behavioral, or systemic interventions" (Gladding, 2018, p. 39). As a higher education professional, you will not likely employ the interventions mentioned in the latter part of the definition, but you will benefit from learning about ways to connect with and empower others. Counseling skills assist in forming a working relationship, listening effectively, and working well with others. A good counselor may also possess other qualities, including warmth, empathy, and open-mindedness, that would be of great benefit to a higher education professional. While you may be tempted to provide immediate advice to students who come to you with concerns, taking the time to listen and allow each student to talk may go a long way toward helping them find their own solutions. Listening skills are critical to forming a productive and empowering relationship with others and can help set the stage for future interactions.

Carl Rogers was a pioneer in the field of counseling, and his influence continues today. He founded person-centered (formerly client-centered) counseling, which employs a nondirective approach, and he identified several characteristics of a counselor that are understood to be essential in the helping process: genuineness, unconditional positive regard, and empathic understanding (Truscott, 2010). Genuineness involves not putting up a professional front, but rather being open to experiencing the moment with clients. The notion of unconditional positive regard involves the counselor accepting clients for who they are. Finally, empathic understanding is fully understanding the subjective world of clients so they feel understood. This empathic understanding must be made known to clients through actions and statements. Rogers believed that most clients have not had the benefit of sensitive, active listening where empathy is provided (Truscott, 2010). In this chapter, we will review the foundational skills for counseling, so that you may be able to employ them in your work with students to engage on a deeper, more understanding level.

Establishing Rapport

There is probably no concept that is more important in counseling than establishing rapport. *Rapport* has been defined as "a warm, personal and trusting relationship" (Gladding, 2018, p. 132), and it is essential to being able to work with others. The first step to helping someone is connecting with them (Mozdzierz et al., 2009), which then allows you to engage with them. Establishing rapport with students begins as soon as you come into contact with them. Being friendly and using a pleasant, inviting tone of voice and manner can assist in building rapport. Other specific behaviors that can assist in building rapport include maintaining eye contact (more about this later) and speaking in an easy, natural voice. Family therapists have long used the concept of *joining*, described as a way to connect with each family member. Joining may be a useful way of connecting with students. Natrajan-Tyagi and Woolley (2017) reported effective joining can also include briefly sharing mutual interests (e.g., "I like soccer too") and sharing general details about yourself ("I also went to college at a large state university"). The goal of joining is to form a safe and trusting connection and remove any reticence the student may have about the encounter. Over time, rapport can be maintained if the helping professional remembers details that the student has shared (e.g., names of family members, important events in the student's life, hobbies or activities).

Listening

Listening may be the most commonly used counseling skill. People want to be listened to and heard. Really listening requires that you concentrate on what the student is sharing and focus solely on that moment. For some students, this may be their first experience of being listened to by a sympathetic and attentive professional.

Listening is often thought to be a passive behavior, with one person actively talking while the other passively takes in what is being communicated (Moursand & Kenny, 2002). However, a good listener is active. Listening requires undivided attention and a nonjudgmental stance. You must listen to the content that is being shared while also noticing how it is being shared. Some people are open about their feelings, but for others, their feelings need to be assessed based on how they present themselves. This type of listening enables the professional to detect what type of emotions individuals are conveying with their comments and behavior (Mozdzierz et al., 2009). Often people will convey their emotions with their behavior. An easy example is the student whose voice begins to rise as he talks about not getting selected as an assistant in the chemistry lab. While he might not have said he is angry, his behavior and vocal tone indicate that he is. Or consider another student, with her head down and tears in her eyes as she says, "I have never been this far away from my family for this long." This statement contains the fact of the student being apart from family, but also conveys feelings that should be addressed, namely homesickness and sadness. A good listener remembers the facts but also identifies the emotions.

Attending

Attending (and listening) skills offer a way for you to make contact with others and hear them accurately (Ivey et al., 2006). These skills include eye contact, tone of voice, and culturally appropriate body language. Taken together, these skills are basic to *empathy*, the ability to be sensitive to and understand the worldview of another person. One way to understand *attending* is to examine the opposite. Have you ever been talking to someone and he appears distracted and looks away? The person is not attending to you. Attending primarily manifests itself in behaviors that show you are listening and following what the person is saying, such as facing them, leaning in a bit toward them, and looking at them while they speak. Of course, when practicing attending behaviors, you must be sensitive to cultural differences. In some cultures, maintaining direct eye contact would be viewed as disrespectful. Perhaps leaning in too close to someone might be interpreted as invading their space. (See Chapter 6 on cultural and diversity awareness for more information.) Students vary in their backgrounds—gender, ethnicity, race, socioeconomic status, religion, sexuality, and a number of other factors. You must be sensitive to these factors, sometimes without even knowing about them. Take, for example, a student who was sexually assaulted in the past. Being alone in a room with a male higher education professional, who begins to lean in toward her, could be perceived as threatening to her.

Attending behaviors also include such actions as a head nod, a "hmmm," or single words or phrases. These are called *encouragers*, or *minimal encouragers*, because they encourage the person to keep talking. They also demonstrate interest on the part of the listener. Ivey et al. (2006) discussed several dimensions of attending behavior. When you talk to someone, you should look at them. You don't want to stare, but look and take natural breaks in eye contact. Using your body language to convey attention is critical. Face the other person and lean in slightly, but with a natural and relaxed manner. You can also demonstrate attending by staying with what has already been said. Remain on the topic that the person has shared; doing so will show the person that you are interested in what they have to say and that you are listening. Have you ever shared an upsetting situation with a friend, and when you were done the friend began to talk about a completely different topic? Chances are you didn't feel listened to or may even have felt that what you shared was not important. Try not to interrupt or change topics when a student is sharing. Carl Rogers described a technique called "simple acceptance" whereby you say, "I see," "Yes," or anything else that lets the person know that they are being heard, followed attentively, understood, and accepted (Kirschenbaum, 2009). Listening to others and not interrupting or sharing your own story communicates that you care and are focused on the person in front of you. Think about a time someone may have listened to you without judgment or interruptions. You likely felt positively about this response.

Minimal encouragers also mean that you as the helper, or listener, provide a minimal response. These can include such words as "go on" or "right." Another type of encourager is to repeat one important word or phrase that the student has just shared (Moursand & Kenny, 2002). For example, the student may say, "I should have known that would happen." Your response might be, "That would happen?" This encourages the student to say more on the topic. You may also use an inviting smile or posture to express interest and encourage the student to keep sharing. One way to encourage students to keep talking is to combine a verbal and nonverbal encourager. So perhaps, in response to the student, you might look directly at them, nod, and say, "Hmm...." These types of minimal encouragers let the student know you are interested and want to hear more.

Asking Questions

If you reflect on any conversation you have had, it likely included a lot of questions. Even typical greetings usually begin with "How are you?" or "What have you been up to?" or "¿Que paso?" or "What's going on?" Using questions is a critical way to gain information from others or to clarify what you have heard. Questions are often designed to move someone from the general to the specific ("When exactly did you start feeling that way?"). But too much reliance on questions can feel like an interrogation, so remember to alternate the counseling skills you use. Questions can also inadvertently guide the direction of the meeting (Moursand & Kenny, 2002). The student may share a lot of information about different topics, but you may ask questions about only one, thus directing the conversation toward that course. Be careful not to rely solely on questions because the student can come to expect this style of interaction and remain silent until you ask one. You don't want to fall into a question-and-answer pattern with the student where you are directing the conversation and the student waits passively for you.

In counseling, questions are often described as either open ended or closed ended. Open-ended questions are used to gain a general picture of a situation (Ivey et al., 1997). These questions include phrases that do not allow the person to reply with only a yes/no or just a few words. Instead, these questions encourage an explanation. Examples include "Tell me about what happened with your roommate" or "What has been going on with that math class?" or "How did that situation come about?" Closed-ended questions are used to obtain facts and specifics. While they help to clarify and provide information, they often lead to short answers. Examples include "Where did you meet him?" or "How often do you skip class?" or "How many people are in the sorority?" Try to avoid questions that require only a yes or no response, since that may be the only reply you get. Your goal is to keep the student talking and providing you with information.

Avoid using questions to make abrupt changes in topic. When a student is sharing, stay on topic. Asking a question about an unrelated topic signals possible disinterest to the student. It also disrupts the flow of the meeting. If you want to change the subject, you could use a summary statement (discussed later in this chapter) to help move the conversation. Ivey et al. (2006) cautioned that asking questions of others may be seen as rude and intrusive for some cultural groups. There is no one set of rules to follow with each group, but being open, honest, and respectful with others goes a long way toward forming a relationship. Pay attention to the student's body language and take your cue from how comfortable or uncomfortable they seem to be with questions.

Reflecting Feeling

A simple way to think about reflection is to imagine a mirror and how it reflects back an image. Reflection in counseling is a technique in which you *reflect* back what the person has just said to you. However, unlike a mirror, you want to change the reflection a bit so you do not sound repetitive. Reflection of *feeling* is intended to lead to more discussion about feelings and verification of feelings (Ivey et al., 1997). Rogers also recommended reflection of feeling but warned that it is difficult to learn (Kirschenbaum, 2009). He cautioned that it requires deep concentration on what the person is saying and then a restatement of what the person has communicated, but with an emphasis on the feeling element. Ultimately, the purpose of the reflection of feeling is to assist the other person in seeing themselves more clearly and objectively. Reflecting feeling involves observing the student's emotions, naming those emotions, and repeating them back to the student (Ivey et al., 2010). For example, "You seem hurt and disappointed that you weren't selected for that scholarship."

The goal of reflection of feeling is that the person will experience and understand their emotional state more fully and talk more deeply about their feelings (Ivey et al., 2010). When engaging in reflection of feeling, you must identify both the spoken and unexpressed feelings. The student's body language and vocal tone may indicate feelings.

Summarizing

The use of summary can be helpful when a person tells you about many things happening in their life and you want to convey that you have been listening. Ivey et al. (1997) described summarization as the way to organize the many facts and feelings of the person and situation. Summarizing is feeding back to the person the essence of longer statements they made. This can include descriptions of behavior, thoughts, and feelings (Ivey et al., 2006).

Summarizing is a great skill to use at the start or end of a meeting. At the start of a meeting, it can be used to restate what was discussed previously with the student: "Amaya, I know the last time I saw you, you were telling me about your roommate and some of her behaviors that offend you. You were struggling to communicate with her." This summary provides the student with the information that was shared to allow her to decide how to begin the conversation. It also shows that you remember what she talked about last time and that it is important to you. Summarizing can also be useful at the end of a meeting to clarify key information that has been shared: "We covered a lot today. Your involvement in the campus ministry and balancing that with your studies. The potential visit from your high school friends and how that is stressing you out a bit. Upcoming midterms and how to handle that one professor who seems to a be a very tough grader. There is a lot going on for you right now."

The use of summary can also be employed during your meeting if you find the student rambling and covering a lot of topics. If you feel a bit lost, it is likely that the student does too. Summarizing can present back to the student all that she has said and allow her to respond on any part of it: "Let me see if I understand what has been going on. You're upset about your parents' divorce and not happy about how they told you. You would like to go home and see your mom, but traveling that far at this point in the semester is impossible. There are a lot of things you need to attend to here at school. It's really hard to prioritize what to do."

Paraphrasing

When you paraphrase what someone says, you are repeating their message back to them to ensure you have heard the facts correctly (Ivey et al., 2006). The idea is not to "parrot," or repeat exactly what the person said, but instead to rephrase it while keeping the main content. Repeating the student's exact words can be frustrating for the student and also not advance the conversation. For example, if the student says, "I am struggling so much with all my classes," you would not want to reply, "You are struggling with all your classes," but rather perhaps, "Your classes are really giving you trouble now." The intent is the same, but the latter response demonstrates a deeper understanding by the listener. The idea of a paraphrase is to add a little something to what the student has shared so that they are encouraged to continue. As another example, if the student shares, "I just have not been able to concentrate on my studies. I find my mind wandering a lot when I sit down to study," an appropriate paraphrase would be, "It's been hard for you to get a lot of studying done. You are not able to concentrate in the way you would like."

Paraphrasing is taking what the student shares with you, building on it, and blending their words with your understanding of what those words mean (Moursand & Kenny, 2002). While this may sound easy, a good paraphrase includes both what is being verbalized and possibly what the student means but has not verbalized. Paraphrases allow the student to hear a restatement of what they shared and know that they have been listened to and heard. It also gives them the chance to correct any misperception on the part of the listener. Sometimes adding a request for correction of your paraphrase can be helpful. For example, adding "Am I hearing you correctly?" or "Is that right?" at the end of a paraphrase allows the student to either agree or disagree (Moursand & Kenny, 2002). Paraphrases lead to verification of facts and thoughts (Ivey et al., 2006).

Although paraphrasing is an important skill, it should not be used in isolation. If the listener relies too heavily on paraphrases, the student may feel stuck or confused. Be careful not to rely on the same introduction to the paraphrase either. You may like phrases such as "Sounds like you are saying..." or "I hear you saying..." or "Seems like you feel as though...." Although these are all excellent choices, you need to vary what you use when working with a student. It's

OK to try a paraphrase with a student and potentially get it wrong. This allows the student to correct you and move on. Don't view this potential correction as a failure on your part; frame it as a way to fully understand what the student is trying to share with you. It is better to be set right by the student ("Well, I don't really feel angry as much as disappointed") than to continue in the misunderstanding. You will be surprised at how forgiving others are when they believe you are trying to listen, help, and understand them.

Responding in a Neutral Manner

An important characteristic of a good counselor is a nonjudgmental stance. Being nonjudgmental means accepting the person in front of you for who they are and what they have to say. This means refraining from a verbal or nonverbal response that might indicate your disagreement or disapproval of the student. It is possible that the student will tell you about behaviors, values, or experiences that you do not agree with or condone. However, you must not vocalize your disagreement; rather, you should listen and let the student talk. This demonstrates acceptance of the student.

Challenges to Your Values

As you work with students, there may be times when they share something that challenges your values. Working with members of a Greek-letter organization, for example, may push your values. While they may be engaged in service to the community, they may also have a reputation for hazing. Or perhaps you have had a family member suffer from substance abuse, and hearing about that level of drunkenness from a student may make you uncomfortable. The standards outlined in *Professional Competency Areas for Student Affairs Educators* encourage higher education professionals to "articulate awareness and understanding of one's attitudes, values, beliefs, assumptions, biases, and identify how they affect one's integrity and work with others" (ACPA–College Student Educators International & NASPA–Student Affairs Administrators in Higher Education, 2015, p. 16). You may not always agree with what the student says, but you do need to show acceptance and support. It is critical to "shelve" your personal values while working with students.

Managing Triggers

Sometimes when a student shares a story or personal issue, it may make you think about something in your own life or remind you of a similar problem you have faced—and it may trigger an emotional reaction in you. *Triggers* are words or actions by another person that spark something in you, typically a negative emotional response. Keeping the focus on the student and their issues, and not expressing your own feelings, is important in remaining supportive and impartial. When listening to a student's problem, higher education professionals must be careful to separate what the student is saying from potential issues in their own life. Professionals may believe they can handle any situation with poise and a neutral response, but this is not always the case. An important part of being a good listener and helper to others is recognizing one's own limitations. Sometimes you will face triggers or issues that are perhaps too close to your own experience to deal with objectively. Take, for example, a student who is sharing with you details about a conflict with a close friend. Your mind may wander to a similar situation you experienced, and it may be hard for you to be objective in your advice. Another example might be a student who is getting tearful over the loss of a parent, which takes you back to your own struggle with the loss of a loved one.

The decision of whether to share your own personal struggle with the student is a controversial issue among helpers. Some advise strictly against it because it takes the focus off the student's issue. The student may feel as though you are telling them to deal with the situation in the same way you did. Alternatively, others believe that showing your own vulnerability or struggle may help the student understand the universality of the issue and also model how to cope effectively. There is no right or wrong way to proceed, and each situation and student may require a different response. Our advice to you as a higher education professional is to make a decision based on what you think will be most helpful to the student and ensure you are not using the student for your own healing.

If you find yourself triggered frequently when working with a particular student, consider seeking help from a colleague in the form of consultation. Talking with a trusted colleague about how you felt when working with the student can help you sort out your reaction. Other ways to manage triggers include developing coping skills you can use when triggers emerge. Coping skills can be grounding techniques (e.g., place feet firmly on the ground, take slow deep breaths) to help you refocus on the student and not your own bodily responses. However, if you find yourself constantly being triggered, you likely have some work to do. You may need to explore your issues in counseling and examine these triggers.

Using Confrontation Cautiously

Skilled and experienced counselors can use confrontation to help a client bring attention to a contradiction in behavior or statements. Ultimately, the goal is to draw the client's awareness to this inconsistency and help them reach a resolution. An example might be a client who is yelling while talking about what happened at work but denies being angry. In this case, the client's behavior and tone of voice imply anger, but the client won't or doesn't want to recognize this feeling. The counselor might say, "You told me that you were not angry about work, but you seem really angry talking about it."

Sometimes when talking to a student, a discrepancy in what they are saying will become obvious. You will be confused and want clarification. However, you must be careful to not sound confrontational. For example, "I thought you said you don't drink at house parties? Seems like you did this weekend." While confrontation is a counseling skill that can be used effectively, it takes some skill and timing; in some cases, it may be best to avoid using this technique. Instead, you may want to clarify something the student says with a question ("I'm sorry, I thought I remember you saying your parents were divorced?"). Your tone of voice in asking the question will probably influence the way the student hears it. Presenting your concern as a confusion rather than a confrontation may help the student reply in a nondefensive manner.

Advice Giving and Problem Solving

While it may be tempting to give advice to others, counselors typically do not engage in this practice. The belief is that, if people are listened to and supported, they can reach their own best decisions. Giving advice raises many problems, including that the student may not follow it. This may leave you surprised or disappointed that your great suggestion was ignored (Ivey et al., 2006). Alternately, the advice you give may have a bad outcome for the student ("Thanks for suggesting I talk to my mentor. He told me to start the project over and get a new idea. Now I am weeks behind."). You may find that many students will be able to solve their problems on their own if you simply listen to them.

One way to avoid advice giving is to think about giving information instead. It's fine to give information—higher education professionals do this commonly in their work. Information giving is letting students know about resources that may be available—for example, telling a student that academic advisors are available on campus to help with course planning. But telling a student that she should go to the academic advisor is advice giving. It's best to say, "Carolina, I am not sure if you know, but academic advisors are available in the student center on the first floor," compared to "You should go to an academic advisor and get that schedule fixed." The former gives information but leaves the decision to utilize the service up to the student. Information empowers students; advice giving can make them dependent on you. A good rule is, if you have the information on hand and the student requests it, you can supply it. If the student asks, "Does the financial aid office take walk-ins?" and you know an appointment is needed, you can simply reply, "I know the office is busy and only takes appointments. They can be made through the student app."

We caution you against solving problems for the student. Your goal should be to empower them to solve their own problems. You can, however, help the student identify the problem they need to solve. Students may be in so much distress that they are unable to determine what the main issues are. Sometimes a student will move from topic to topic and the session may begin to appear as though it is falling apart. This may be the time to use a summary statement and try to focus the student on the main issues. It is not the time to jump in and try to solve any of the student's problems.

Advice giving *may* be appropriate when the student is dealing with a crisis (Moursand & Kenny, 2002). There may be times when the student does not seem to be thinking rationally or responsibly. Take the example of a student who seems to be getting more ill every day. You could say, "I am concerned about your health and the symptoms you have been exhibiting. I think you may want to seek medical help if this continues much longer." This statement both shows your concern and provides some advice. This is in stark contrast to saying, "You should drop that class. I don't think you will be able to pull up your grade this term." The latter statement is disrespectful and unkind, and it implies you know what is best for the student.

Conclusion

When you first begin to work with students in a professional role, you may feel overwhelmed, uncertain about how to reply, and at a loss for words. These are natural feelings that many higher education professionals have at the start of their career. Over time and with more experience, you will become skilled at responding to anything students tell you. You will also develop your own personal style of helping and listening that will be congruent with who you are as a person and comfortable for you to implement. You will develop a range of skills that you can draw on. Think of these skills as tools in your box; you will need to use more than one with each student.

It is important to instill hope in students that their condition will improve, but also help them remain realistic. You want to be optimistic with students about their situations so that they believe some resolution can be found. However, it is not a good idea to promise results or minimize a serious condition. Recognizing each of these situations can be tricky. You may want to say, "I know you are a bright and competent student and I think you will find a solution to this problem" to lift up the student so that they can feel motivated and positive. Conversely, if the predicament of the student is very serious, as you will see in subsequent chapters, you must not falsely promise solutions. For example, a student who is depressed and has perhaps turned to drugs as a way of coping should not be told that things will get better. Things may get better, or things may get worse. When working with students such as this, it is best to say, "Things are really rough for you right now. It feels as though there is no good way out. I am concerned about you and think getting some professional help is a good way to start." This statement shows some optimism about the student getting help but also does not promise that things will improve. You do not want to say, "Things are looking bleak now, but I am sure you will snap out of this down mood." Issues such as depression and substance abuse are not easily "fixed," and the student will likely need professional help to manage or overcome these issues.

References

ACPA–College Student Educators International & NASPA–Student Affairs Administrators in Higher Education. (2015). *Professional competency areas for student affairs educators.* https://www.naspa.org/images/uploads/main/ACPA_NASPA_Professional_Competencies_FINAL.pdf

Gladding, S. (2018). *The counseling dictionary* (4th ed.). American Counseling Association.

Ivey, A. E., Bradford Ivey, M., & Zalaquett, C. P. (2010). *Intentional interviewing and counseling* (7th ed.). Cengage Learning.

Ivey, A. E., Packard, N. G., & Ivey, M. (2006). *Basic attending skills* (4th ed.). Microtraining Associates.

Ivey, A. E., Packard, N. G., & Ivey, M. (1997). *Basic influencing skills* (3rd ed.). Microtraining Associates.

Kirschenbaum, H. (2009). *The life and work of Carl Rogers.* American Counseling Association.

Moursand, J., & Kenny, M. (2002). *The process of counseling and therapy* (4th ed.). Prentice Hall.

Mozdzierz, G., Peluso, P., & Lisiecki, J. (2009). *Principles of counseling and psychotherapy: Learning essential domains and nonlinear thinking of master practitioners.* Routledge.

Natrajan-Tyagi, R., & Woolley, S. R. (2017). Joining in couple and family therapy. In J. Lebow, A. Chambers, & D. Breunlin (Eds.), *Encyclopedia of couple and family therapy.* Springer, Cham. https://doi.org/10.1007/978-3-319-15877-8_564-1

Truscott, D. (2010). *Becoming an effective psychotherapist: Adopting a theory of psychotherapy that's right for you and your client.* American Psychological Association.

CHAPTER 3

Setting Boundaries and Understanding Confidentiality

Because higher education professionals often develop close relationships with students, they are in a strategic position to intervene when students find themselves in crisis. The challenge, however, is that such professionals do not serve in a clinical role and thus are not under the same restrictions as counselors in a counseling center. Although nonclinical professionals are not bound by the Health Insurance Portability and Accountability Act of 1996 (HIPAA), certain standard ethical practices nevertheless must be considered. Often this ethical area is one of concern for both the student and the staff member—this not knowing exactly the correct protocols in handling sensitive information. The Family Educational Rights and Privacy Act (FERPA) presents another area of confusion, as it is an often-misunderstood piece of legislation. This chapter will review the basics of FERPA and how it applies to working with students in crisis. The chapter will also discuss the Clery Act and mandatory reporting. An important skill for professionals to develop is knowing how to uphold institutional protocols while still supporting students in crisis. The chapter will examine the importance of balancing the role of supportive staff member while not crossing personal boundaries—and how to achieve such balance in an empathic and caring way.

Boundaries and Confidentiality

By nature of their roles, higher education professionals are often in a position where students may feel comfortable disclosing personal information. Those professionals who have truly embraced the philosophy of *in loco parentis*, which literally means "in the place of parents," are able to develop deep connections with their students. Those students see them as parental or as an older sibling figure and will often turn to them with serious personal problems. At the same time, higher education professionals will often be the first ones to notice when a student is struggling or when something seems off. They will approach the student to ask what's going on, encouraging the student to discuss the matter. While this outreach is all positive and encouraged, it raises the issue of confidentiality and setting appropriate boundaries. Borshuk (2017) talked about her experience in the classroom, where she sets up important expectations as faculty member. She discusses the importance of being clear about her role as a teacher, not a licensed clinical psychologist. She reminds her students that because she is a teacher, there is no expectation of privacy or confidentiality. This approach creates a safe space for sharing but also sets clear boundaries and expectations; it can be applied to non-classroom settings too. As students feel comfortable with self-disclosure, it is important to remind them of the parameters.

Similar issues are raised with residential staff, such as resident assistants and residence hall directors. These staff members, living alongside their students, naturally develop close bonds. This proximity can pose a challenge when residential staff hear sensitive or concerning information. Students sometimes raise serious mental health concerns, however, and the question is always about what level of confidentiality they should expect—and at what point the staff member is obligated to report the conversation to the institution (Canto et al., 2017). To start, higher education professionals must possess some understanding of HIPAA and FERPA. Both acts will be discussed further in this chapter. Although the laws do provide some guidance, they can be complicated and murky—and can vary in interpretation.

Despite the parameters of these laws, higher education professionals still need to find ways to have positive interactions with their students when discussing these sensitive issues. It is not easy for a student to choose to disclose very personal details, and this act of disclosure is an important step toward getting comfort and help. It is such a tricky balance—wanting to both provide a welcoming and safe environment for open discussion and remain transparent about possible required next steps and disclosures.

Developing Relationships

The most positive relationships between students and administrators exist when there is a healthy balance between the personal and the professional. Administrators must exercise their best judgment when building rapport and establishing these connections, as such relationships can be very beneficial for students and staff members alike. Higher education professionals can develop appropriate relationships in a variety of ways that maintain effective, professional boundaries. One way is to know students by name and story. Administrators can engage in certain behaviors, such as humor, eye contact, informal conversation, and self-disclosure when relevant and appropriate. Getting to know students on a personal level helps develop rapport and lets students know that the higher education professional is invested in them as people. It also increases students' comfort level and willingness to share stories and struggles.

Often in difficult situations, letting students know up front that it might not be possible to offer full confidentiality can be helpful. When it becomes clear that the student is dealing with a sensitive or personal issue, it can sometimes help to let them know that if they need an assurance of confidentiality, they might want to consider the counseling center. Saying something like, "I am here to listen and support you, but I am bound to some different rules than those of the counselors. While I will always do whatever I can to maintain your privacy, if you feel you need full confidentiality in what you'd like to share with me, you might want to consider talking to someone in the counseling center." That way, students know at the outset their limits and boundaries in sharing.

Laws, Regulations, and Privacy

Given how closely higher education professionals work with students, there will inevitably be moments when it becomes difficult to know where to draw the line regarding privacy. It is important for higher education professionals to have a basic understanding of the laws and regulations surrounding confidentiality, privacy, and reporting. Although these administrators need not be experts in the details of each law or regulation, they should have at least some level of knowledge so as to avoid potentially problematic situations. We will discuss the basic laws and regulations, but higher education professionals should familiarize themselves with any additional expectations and protocols at their own institutions.

FERPA

In 1974, New York Senator James Buckley created a bill that would protect the rights of students. His efforts resulted in the Family Educational Rights and Privacy Act (FERPA), or, as it is often called, the Buckley Amendment. It can be challenging to interpret what the original intent of this legislation was, as it lacks the extensive and traditional legislative history of other laws and amendments (Schulze, 2009). The Supreme Court case of *Gonzaga University v. Doe* found that a student could not sue under this act. As a result, there are few judicial interpretations of FERPA, leaving higher education professionals to rely on "Dear Colleague" letters from the Family Policy Compliance Office of the U.S. Department of Education (DOE, 2016). These texts can be helpful in clarifying the legislation's language and intent.

Over the years, Congress has amended FERPA's language several times, and the DOE has worked to clarify the regulations governing the interpretation of FERPA. It remains, however, one of the most misunderstood, confusing, and misused regulations in higher education. When administrators are dealing with issues of boundaries and confidentiality, FERPA only adds to the level of stress and concern. With all its rules, interpretations, and exceptions, the legislation still often remains confusing and murky at best.

FERPA's (1974) regulations pertain to "educational records." This is one of the biggest areas of confusion. What, exactly, is an "educational record"? Under FERPA, an *educational record* is defined as records, files, documents, and other materials that contain information directly related to a student. These records are maintained by an educational agency or institution or by a person acting on behalf of the agency or institution. FERPA's main goal is to limit access to student records to all but the student. Exceptions exist, and, when they are understood correctly, can help higher education professionals do their jobs effectively and with sensitivity. Institutions are allowed to release information to school officials, including faculty, who demonstrate a legitimate educational interest in the student. In other words, there has to be an educational reason determined in order to gain access to the records. In these cases, educational records can be released without consent. Parents hold the rights for students under age 18, and the institution can release a student's records when parents have given a written consent for such release. Once students reach age 18, their parents can no longer access their records—except in cases where the child is a tax dependent. When students are financially dependent on their parents, as defined in section 152 of the Internal Revenue Code of 1986, campus officials may disclose all student education record information to parents (34 CFR § 99.31). This exception to FERPA regulations allows each institution to create its own set of protocols for disclosing information to parents, without having to rely on the health emergency exception.

There are base guidelines to which every school must adhere in order to remain in compliance with FERPA. Many institutions go well above and beyond these requirements, creating an extra cushion of protection. Higher education professionals must ensure they understand the expectations of their institutions so that they act accordingly and within the guidelines and expectations set for them.

Mandatory Reporting and the Clery Act

Along with FERPA, the Clery Act is another piece of legislation that can cause concern and confusion for higher education professionals. Knowing what and when to report an incident is an important step in setting up appropriate and safe boundaries.

After a Lehigh University student was murdered in her dorm room in 1986, her parents spearheaded efforts in 1990 to create the Jeanne Clery Disclosure of Campus Security Policy and Campus Crime Statistics Act, which is named in her memory. The intent of this federal act is to protect students by requiring colleges and universities to be transparent about crimes that occur on campus. College administrators must report all serious criminal allegations made to them "in good faith" to a designated campus official. "Good faith" is defined as beyond just rumors. The campus official reports these allegations to the DOE. In turn, these campus crime statistics are published each year for every school in the country that receives federal financial aid, which is almost all of them. It is important to note that campus officials are required to report only that a crime occurred, not any personal information. This is a crucial distinction. When talking to students in crisis, higher education professionals can explain that while they might be required to report that a crime has been committed, they do not need to divulge the victim's personal or identifying information.

To remain compliant with the Clery Act, all colleges and universities that receive federal funding must distribute a public annual security report (ASR) to all employees and students by October 1. This report must include statistics of campus crime for the preceding 3 calendar years. ASRs must also describe any efforts taken to improve safety on their campuses and include policy statements regarding (but not limited to) crime reporting, campus facility security and access, law enforcement authority, incidence of alcohol and drug use, and the prevention of/response to sexual assault, domestic or dating violence, and stalking.

Conclusion

The bottom line is that this area of higher education administration is complicated. On the one hand, higher education professionals are often in the best position to have meaningful and helpful conversations about sensitive and personal information. On the other hand, this level of comfort can put that faculty or staff member in a tough position if the student discloses information that requires reporting, or if the student begins to rely on them to an extent that becomes unhealthy or unproductive, or both.

Knowing the laws and regulations, as well as specific institutional expectations and protocols, will help the higher education professional with these interactions—enabling open and honest conversations and allowing both students and professionals to understand how the conversation will go and any next steps that might need to be taken. The key here is balancing the legal and ethical obligations while still supporting the student. Higher education professionals must maintain professional boundaries as they give comfort and help to their students. This work is not easy, but understanding the applicable laws—and how to create a safe, appropriate space for students—will allow for an even more successful outcome for all involved.

References

Borshuk, C. (2017, February). Managing student self-disclosure in class settings: Lessons from feminist pedagogy. *Journal of the Scholarship of Teaching and Learning, 17*(1), 78–86. https://doi.org/10.14434/v17i1.20070

Canto, A., Cox, B., Hayden, S., Becker, M., & Osborn, D. (2017). College students in crisis: Prevention, identification, and response options for campus housing professionals. *The Journal of College and University Student Housing, 43*(2), 44–57.

Family Policy Compliance Office, U.S. Department of Education. (2016, August 24). *Dear colleague letter to school officials at institutions of higher education.* https://studentprivacy.ed.gov/sites/default/files/resource_document/file/DCL_Medical%20Records_Final%20Signed_dated_9-2.pdf

Family Educational Rights and Privacy Act of 1974, 20 U.S.C. § 1232(g) (2020). https://www.govinfo.gov/content/pkg/USCODE-2020-title20/pdf/USCODE-2020-title20-chap31-subchapIII-part4-sec1232g.pdf

Jeanne Clery Disclosure of Campus Security Policy and Campus Crime Statistics Act of 1990, 20 U.S.C. §1092(f) (2020). https://www.govinfo.gov/content/pkg/USCODE-2020-title20/pdf/USCODE-2020-title20-chap28-subchapIV-partG-sec1092.pdf

Schulze, L. N. (2009). Balancing law student privacy interests and progressive pedagogy: Dispelling the myth that FERPA prohibits cutting-edge academic support methodologies. *Widener Law Journal, 19,* 215–253. https://ecollections.law.fiu.edu/faculty_publications/223

CHAPTER 4

Stages of Change and Making Referrals

This chapter will cover the important skill of determining how and when higher education professionals need to make an appropriate referral to counseling centers on campus or, in some instances, off-campus services. Often students will develop a trusting relationship with a staff member, confide in them, and continue to seek them out for assistance and guidance. This chapter will explain how and when to make a successful referral to counseling as well as what to expect from counseling and how to support students once a referral has been made. The chapter will also discuss Prochaska's (1979) stages of change model and motivational interviewing, and how both can affect students' decisions to seek help.

Making a Change: Prochaska's Stages of Change Model

Deciding to make a change is not easy. Take a moment to think about it. What does that process look like? Do people just wake up one day and make a change? This is highly unlikely. For most people, change is a gradual process. It needs to be thought about, planned, and ultimately executed. The same is true for students. If students are struggling with an issue, perhaps personal or academic, higher education professionals may see the signs and recognize the need for change long before students are ready to do so themselves. Change is a process. Prochaska's (1979) stages of change model can clarify how students might approach taking the steps needed to acknowledge their behavior and move toward active and engaged behavioral change.

In Stage 1, *precontemplation*, students are still in denial that there even is a problem with their behavior. For example, they might say something like, "I don't have a problem with drinking. Everyone blacks out now and then. Besides, most of my friends drink twice as much as I do." In this stage, it would be most helpful to focus on expressing concern about particular behaviors, to raise their awareness of the issue. A helpful response would be something like, "I worry about what might happen to you when you're blacked out. You also seem to be drinking a lot more than you used to and missing more classes." This response will help students start to see that their behavior has consequences.

In Stage 2, students have moved into *contemplation*. This stage is exactly like it sounds; students will start to engage in an internal debate about the existence or significance of their problem. Their behavior may appear very inconsistent. In this stage, they might say, "I know I should talk to someone in counseling about my panic attacks; it's just that I don't have time. Besides, I'm sure they're really busy with people with more important problems." Higher education professionals can help students talk through both sides of the concern. Be careful not to push them, as this may increase their resistance. Try responding with, "Your panic attacks seem to really be getting in the way this week. I know how busy you are though. It must seem impossible to fit anything else in." Using this type of technique will help students engage in self-reflection and encourage them to contemplate both sides of their issue.

Stage 3 is *preparation*. At this stage, students are committed to change and will begin to make plans to follow through. As the name of the stage suggests, students will begin to prepare themselves to make the desired change. They might say something like, "I'm going to go and talk to someone at the counseling center about my sleep problems. The center is only open in the day though, and that's when I've been sleeping lately." In this stage, higher education professionals can help by supporting the planning process. Try suggesting something like, "I know the counseling center is open Wednesday evenings; why don't we call right now and see if you can get an appointment then. I'll go with you." The goal is always to help students move from one stage of the model to the next.

In Stage 4, students are ready for *action*. They have taken steps to address the problem and are ready to begin to make a change. In this stage, students might say things like, "I've been seeing a counselor and she says I should be getting out of my room more instead of avoiding others to control my social anxiety." Higher education professionals can support students' follow-through. Help them with this step by saying, "I know how hard it is for you to go to the cafeteria. How about I meet you there for lunch tomorrow at noon?" This type of reinforcement can help students move through this stage.

The final stage is *maintenance*. At this stage, students have successfully moved through the previous four stages and are at the point where they are ready to maintain changes until the behaviors become habitual. This might be a statement like, "Exercising has really helped improve my mood and energy; it's just with finals coming up next week I'm not sure I'll have time to get to the gym." It is important to help support the changes students have made to this point. Higher education professionals can acknowledge students' concerns while also offering support to help them maintain their progress. Try saying, "I can see how that's stressful. Managing time can be tough. Why don't you make a pact with a friend to go together at least on Tuesday and Thursday of next week?"

Motivational Interviewing

Along with understanding the process of how people change, it can be helpful to know a bit about motivational interviewing (MI). This will allow for a smoother conversation when trying to encourage students to take action. This technique is a more clinical method but can be adapted for use by higher education professionals when trying to help students find the intrinsic motivation and commitment needed for real and sustained change. MI is based on the person and centered around goals, with the focus on creating a real sense of internal motivation and commitment (Miller & Rollnick, 2002). One of the main components of MI is using OARS: asking open-ended questions (O), affirming (A), reflecting (R), and summarizing (S). These skills were discussed in Chapter 2 and are useful to apply when using MI. Empathy is another essential skill when using MI, to show students you understand what they are going through. Using these skills will help students find their own reasons for change, which is the real purpose of MI: to get students to come to their own realizations and goals for wanting to act. When using MI, help students focus on four categories: desire, ability, reasons, and need. As they work through each of these categories, students will increase their commitment to making long-lasting change (Miller & Moyers, 2006). When talking with students, it is key to avoid direct opposition to their thinking, which could reinforce resistance. For example, a student thinking about their relationship might say, "I don't have a problem with my relationship. Maybe we fight too much sometimes, but it's not a big deal." They are expressing resistance to change. Countering with a statement like, "You seem to have a problem based on what I have seen, and you need to break up immediately" is likely to reinforce that resistance. Perhaps try something more thought-provoking, like, "So, you fight too much at times, but you haven't really experienced any negative consequences or had any problems as a result. Is that how you feel?" A good next question once students seem open to making a change might be, "OK, so what's next?" This allows students to begin to visualize exactly what making this change might look like in their life.

Things to Consider When Reaching Out

Knowing the Prochaska (1979) model and the basics of MI provides a strong foundation for understanding how people approach and commit to making a change in their life. It also helps to understand when someone is not ready for change and to view that as part of the process. Having a good sense of how to approach students when there is a concern will encourage movement toward positive change. The strategies discussed in this chapter can help ensure that this is a positive interaction. The relationships higher education professionals develop with students are important. People are more willing to listen to and take advice from those they feel close to and with whom they have developed a relationship (MacGeorge et al., 2008). Developing these relationships and building trust begins long before a student needs help.

When you want to intervene after noticing a problem, make sure there is enough time for a full discussion. It is important not to rush this discussion in between meetings or when the student needs to be elsewhere. Be mindful of privacy. If you're in a highly visible office or a high-traffic area where the student might not feel comfortable speaking openly, consider meeting somewhere else. Maybe ask the student where they would like to meet.

During these conversations, remember to use empathy as much as possible. Using supportive language like, "It's hard to make a change. You've been doing this for so long, it probably feels like you could never stop" will help students feel understood and not judged. Telling students what to do or trying to fix their problem will be less effective than really listening and understanding their struggles. When students feel heard, they will be more likely to respond.

Magic Number Theory

Helping others to make a positive change can be frustrating. At times it may seem as though all your attempts to help students have no effect. It is important to keep in mind that everyone changes at their own pace and when they are ready. Talking with students and pointing out their behavior is an important step in their journey to making a change. There's an idea that everyone has a *magic number* of encounters they need before they will commit to making a change—in other words, they need to hear from a certain number of people about their concerning behaviors and recommendations that they get some help before they finally say to themselves, "Maybe it is actually time I seek support and get the help I need to make some changes in my life." No one knows their own number, and no one knows what number they are on another person's journey. But someone must be the first. Keep this in mind if a student politely says "thank you" and chooses not to seek help. Maybe they just haven't reached their magic number yet. But the conversation almost certainly moved them one step closer.

When to Make a Referral

One of the most challenging issues in helping students is knowing when to make a referral to counseling. Students will develop relationships with higher education professionals and come to rely on them. But there will come a time when a referral to counseling makes sense. When the higher education professional feels they cannot help anymore or the problem is beyond their scope, it will be time to refer the student. A referral is also necessary if there is a concern for the student's health or safety. You can reassure students that plenty of others need help and that is why the counseling center exists. Some students may have been raised to keep family business inside the family and not talk to outsiders. Some may have cultural views that do not support seeking counseling. Others may feel that talking won't help. Still others may feel seeking help is a sign of weakness or being crazy. Be prepared to discuss these beliefs with students. Alternatively, while students might be aware of the services available, they may not feel confident that these services will help, or they may have concerns about the stigma associated with going to the counseling center (Eisenberg et al., 2007). Reducing these stigmas and continuing to remove barriers will go a long way toward increasing students' use of counseling on campus.

A critical skill for higher education professionals is understanding and recognizing the difference between a student in distress and student in crisis. When a student is in distress, it is usually a result of stress that has built up over time, and they have had trouble managing it until it eventually came to a head (Swanbrow Becker & Drum, 2015). If this seems to be the case, the best approach is to help the student identify the source of the stress and encourage them to find ways to develop more effective coping strategies. A student in crisis, by contrast, is usually triggered by a single event or circumstance that puts them in a situation where their coping skills cannot respond to and manage the sudden trauma (Swanbrow Becker & Drum, 2015). This is when higher education professionals need to use a more direct approach and refer the student to the counseling center for more immediate attention.

Being an available and knowledgeable resource can make a big difference. Students need guidance in finding the appropriate resources and help; often it is not lack of desire but lack of information that stops them from seeking aid (Eisenberg et al., 2007). Before you have a conversation about referral with students, make sure to familiarize yourself with your campus' support services. Know what campus resources are available for additional support and have this information ready to share. Students may ask what will happen if they choose to go to the counseling center. Be ready to answer that question. Know what happens in a counseling session and be able to discuss the nature and importance of confidentiality, as this is often something students have questions and concerns about. In cases where more intensive help is needed than can be offered at the campus counseling center, be ready to support outside options for treatment and help, as these might be suggested by the counseling center.

Knowing how the counseling process is structured will also help in making the referral. Each campus has its own protocols and procedures on scheduling appointments, limits on how many each student can have, and fee structures. Most campuses offer free, confidential counseling, but sessions are not always unlimited, and depending on the demand, there could be a slight wait time to be seen. If a student seems open to counseling but is hesitating, offer to pick up the phone and help schedule the appointment, or even offer to walk with them to the counseling center to make the appointment. It can also be helpful for a higher education professional to have an established relationship with members of the counseling center team. That way, when making the referral it becomes easier to say, "I know them over there, and they are so nice. Why don't I call my friend George directly and see what we can get set up for you?"

Always remember to follow up. Often the hardest part of the work for students is after they have begun attending counseling. Be sure to check in with the student to see how they are doing and to continue offering support. Remind them that counseling can be hard work. Just as they have to study for school, they may need to put in time for counseling, both in and outside of the sessions.

Conclusion

Students will often be reluctant to seek help on their own due to barriers, stigma, and lack of information. Higher education professionals are in a position to break down these walls and help increase access to professional help. Knowing how change happens, understanding the best ways to approach these conversations, and being aware of resources available are key elements in helping students. Understanding the differences between normal stress and crisis will also help higher education professionals know when it is appropriate to step in and make a referral to counseling. Sometimes students just need a supportive person to listen to them; other times, they need the guidance of a more skilled professional. Knowing that difference is important. As higher education professionals develop confidence in their own knowledge and abilities, they will be better able to support their students.

References

Eisenberg, D., Golbertein, E., & Gollust, S. (2007). Help-seeking and access to mental health care in a university student population. *Medical Care, 45*(7), 594–601. https://doi.org/10.1097/mlr.0b013e31803bb4c1

MacGeorge, E. L., Feng, B., & Thompson, E. R. (2008). "Good" and "bad" advice: How to advise more effectively. In M. Motley (Ed.), *Applied interpersonal communication: Behaviors that affect outcomes* (pp. 145–164). Thousand Oaks, CA: Sage

Miller, W., & Moyers, T. (2006). Eight stages in learning motivational interviewing. *Journal of Teaching in the Addictions, 5*(1), 3–17. https://doi.org/10.1300/J188v05n01_02

Miller, W. R., & Rollnick, S. (2002). *Motivational interviewing: Preparing people for change* (2nd ed.). Guilford Press.

Prochaska, J. O. (1979). *Systems of psychotherapy: A transtheoretical analysis.* Dorsey.

Swanbrow Becker, M., & Drum, D. (2015). Essential counseling knowledge and skills to prepare student affairs staff to promote emotional wellbeing and to intervene with students in distress. *Journal of College & Character, 16*(4), 201–208. https://doi.org/10.1080/2194587X.2015.1091363

CHAPTER 5

Self-Care

This chapter will emphasize the importance of self-care for the higher education professional. Professionals need to practice good nutrition, exercise, diet, recreation, relaxation, and stress management, which are all avenues that help promote self-care. The main focus of these strategies helps professionals find an appropriate work–life balance. The chapter will review wellness and other positive actions that promote one's physical, emotional, and spiritual well-being, as well as examine the concept of resiliency for higher education professionals. Burnout is another important topic to discuss, as professionals may become too attached to their work or the students they help and may suffer from feelings of helplessness and dissolution. This chapter will cover methods to manage stress and ward off burnout, as well as ways to maintain resiliency and remain strong in the face of adversity.

The Higher Education Professional's Work

Work is part of one's identity and can bring great satisfaction. Higher education professionals' work involves daily contact with primarily young adults who are in an exciting stage of their life. They are committed to learning, athletics, arts, student government, and a wide range of social activities. Their outlook and perspective can be refreshing and motivating. However, these same students may be experiencing a number of anxieties and problems due to their stage of life, family circumstances, student status, or more serious mental health concerns. The issues that the students are dealing with may begin to weigh on the professionals with whom they interact. The work of higher education professionals requires attention, care, concern, and an understanding of the unique needs of various subpopulations of students (e.g., LGBTQIA+ students, athletes, international students, nontraditional students such as older-aged students and students returning to college after a career). In addition to responding to student needs, higher education professionals are faced with other demands on their workday, such as attending meetings and meeting deadlines. At times, professionals may begin to feel overwhelmed. The same work that can bring satisfaction, engagement, and fulfillment can also take its toll. Changes in the work environment over the past decade have burdened professionals with heavy workloads and with work "overflow" outside working hours (Poulsen et al., 2014). By the end of a semester or academic year, higher education professionals may feel depleted. Every aspect of their work, along with the myriad skills they must employ, can contribute to feelings of stress and potentially burnout.

Stress is a part of everyone's life, and higher education professionals are no exception. Managing stress is the key to good mental and physical health. Achieving balance in your personal and professional life and managing the demands of the job are necessary to function most effectively and be happy.

Stress

An estimated 80% of Americans experience stress (Werneburg et al., 2018); it can manifest itself in both physical and emotional symptoms such as headaches, feeling overwhelmed, nervousness, anxiety, sadness, or depression (American Psychological Association, 2017). There are different forms of stress, such as acute and chronic. Acute stress is experienced for a short period of time. Perhaps you are in the middle of purchasing a new car and have to contend with a lot of details—loans, insurance, maintenance packages—and you're concerned about how it will all work out. This stress is likely to end after the car is purchased. But chronic stress can be related to situations that are not likely to change, such as caring for an elderly relative with dementia or being in a conflictual and unrewarding marriage. Workplace stress is a common form of stress (Taylor, 2020) and it can become chronic if you are in a job that does not make you happy. The stress you experience in these situations does not diminish and may harm your mental and physical health.

Stress affects the immune system primarily by weakening it (Taylor, 2020). People under stress show increased rates of infectious diseases and colds as well as mononucleosis. Continued exposure to stressful situations poses a risk to health because of high cardiovascular activation (e.g., elevated heart rate, hypertension) as well as chronic sleep difficulties (Taylor, 2020). Exposure to chronic stress can, at times, lead people to use maladaptive coping mechanisms, such as alcohol and drugs, poor diet, and unhealthy sleep habits. All of these coping mechanisms can contribute to the development of other medical conditions. The best way to deal with stress is to recognize when you are experiencing it and find ways to manage your reaction to it. In the case of experiencing temporary feelings of stress, such as a work deadline, these feelings are likely to go away once the deadline is met. However, managing chronic stress is critical to maintaining a healthy life.

Positive coping strategies may buffer the effects of stress. One healthy way to decrease stress is to socialize (Cohen & Janicki-Devartis, 2009). Socialization has the added benefit of boosting the immune system and warding off depression. Schueller and Parks (2014) suggested that increasing the amount of social contact one has as well as the quality of one's interpersonal relationships are both pathways to happiness. So, the next time you need to relieve stress, push yourself away from your desk and join friends for a night out. Create a book club, take a walk outside in nature with others, or enjoy a sporting activity with friends. If you live on campus, it is particularly important to find outlets separate from your on-campus life. Think about your support system and who you can lean on during tough times. What friend can you call? Who is a good listener for you? Gaining the emotional support of friends and family while dealing with a stressful situation helps. Other ways to manage stress include getting enough sleep, eating a healthy diet, and exercising regularly. If you are experiencing chronic stress and these interventions are not helping, you may need a mental health professional to assist you in a stress reduction plan. Strategies may include using a log to monitor your stress and identify the stressful events in your life, practicing muscle relaxation, managing negative self-talk, and attending time management and assertiveness training. These strategies can all be implemented with a helping professional to assist in stress reduction (Barlow et al., 2018).

Burnout

Herbert Freudenberger (1974) coined the term *burnout* to describe the consequences of severe stress in the helping professions. He described burnout as a "feeling of exhaustion and fatigue" (p. 160). Burnout can occur when a professional no longer has the energy for their work. Corey et al. (2019) stated that if professionals are not adequately prepared, "they may be especially vulnerable to early disenchantment, distress and burnout due to unrealistic expectations" (p. 58). Professionals can feel overly responsible for the students they work with, take their work home, and begin to feel overwhelmed by their responsibilities. The working conditions (e.g., long hours, low pay), nature of the work (e.g., student contact, demand for accountability), and high expectations of "face time" all likely contribute to high burnout and attrition rates in the field of higher education and student affairs. An estimated 50% to 60% of new professionals leave the field within the first 5 years of their careers (Tull, 2006).

Working in human service fields has been found to be strongly associated with burnout—specifically the organizational culture of the work environment, with low reward and low support for a highly demanding position. Higher education professionals are often the first people students turn to when they have a problem. Although higher education professionals are not counselors, they respond to students with empathy. At times, this connection can lead to the professional feeling anxious or stressed and taking on the student's concerns.

Burnout can compromise a person's physical health; increase their risk of mental health issues, including depression; and lead to poor job performance, absenteeism from work, substance abuse, and low self-esteem (Maslach & Leiter, 2016). Maslach (2003) described burnout as a job-related stress that results in the professional feeling physically and emotionally exhausted and experiencing little personal accomplishment. Corey et al. (2019) warned that if professionals do not deal with feelings of burnout, they may become impaired, leaving them unable to function at their job.

When a person experiences burnout in the workplace, it is often the result of a mismatch between the individual and the work environment (DuBois & Mistretta, 2020). Leiter and Maslach (2008) identified six domains of the workplace environment that contribute to burnout, including workload, individual's perception of administrative and organizational fairness, lack of control, insufficient reward, conflict between personal and organizational values, and breakdown of community. Individual qualities and characteristics also contribute to how someone handles stress, which may explain why one person develops burnout while another does not (DuBois & Mistretta, 2020). Individuals who have developed healthy coping skills may respond better to stress and thus reduce the likelihood of burnout.

In their 7-year longitudinal study, Hakanen and Schaufeli (2012) found that burnout predicted depressive symptoms and not vice versa. Their results support the hypothesis that work-related well-being spills over to general, context-free well-being. More specifically, burnout and work engagement predict depressive symptoms and life satisfaction over time. This longitudinal study shows that work engagement may have positive consequences for health and well-being. It seems the positive effects of work engagement go beyond the negative impact of burnout, which suggests that work can also benefit one's general well-being. This means that if you are satisfied with your job, these "good" feelings will affect your general well-being.

Barkhuizen et al. (2014) found that the academics in their study who experienced high levels of job demands were likely to develop high levels of burnout, which, in turn, led to health problems. Burnout does not occur in the first months on the job; it may take years to develop. But just as it takes time to develop, it may also take time to recover from it. Pryce et al. (2007) reported that the worker may have to leave the work environment to recover from burnout. If it is not possible for the worker to change their work environment or culture, then they should aim to change where and with whom they work (Pryce et al., 2007).

Have you ever experienced signs of burnout? If so, how did you know you were getting burned out? Intense feelings of disconnectedness from your work, constant tension, sleep difficulties, excessive worry about work, and other effects on your general health (e.g., headaches, fatigue) can all be signs of burnout. Drinking too much alcohol can also be a sign of burning out. Turning to substances may initially feel good and take mental focus off work demands. However, over time, dependence can develop, and performance at work, and elsewhere, may be impaired. Other signs of burnout can be overeating ("stress eating"), frequently calling in sick to work, putting off work tasks until they pile up, or experiencing irritability at work.

One way to help ward off burnout is to engage in a "wind-down ritual" (MacKay, 2020). This process is practiced after work to decompress and disconnect. Experts recommend detaching from the workday by removing work devices from view (e.g., put away your laptop and reports). Spend some time alone to recover from the social demands of work and home. Engage in an enjoyable and challenging hobby. Some individuals also find that following a closing ritual for the workday helps to detach, such as closing all the work browsers on their computer or removing files or other papers from view or stacking them neatly. Later in the chapter, we will examine other self-care strategies that can help with warding off burnout.

Resiliency

Although we have reviewed some potential hazards of working in higher education, it is equally critical to examine ways in which professionals can be proactive in ensuring that the stressors and demands of work and life do not overwhelm them. Developing resilience in the face of pressures and adverse life events is one way to achieve a satisfying and productive life, both at work and at home. Werneburg et al. (2018) defined *resiliency* as "the ability to manage and grow throughout life's challenges" (p. 45). Robertson and Cooper (2013) proposed a multidimensional model of resilience that includes four components: adaptability (flexibility and adapting to changing situations), confidence (feelings of competence and effectiveness), purposefulness (having a clear sense of purpose), and social support (good relationships with others).

Resilience is often described as "hardiness," "resourcefulness," or "mental toughness" (Corey & Corey, 2021). Resilience is frequently used to refer to an individual who has not only survived a difficult situation but is also thriving. Why some crumble in the time of crisis and others respond and adapt may be related to their resilience. Some who are faced with a traumatic event emerge with newfound strength and self-confidence in their ability to cope (Muratori & Haynes, 2020). While we are not suggesting that working in higher education is traumatic, aspects of the work may expose professionals to traumatic material from students, and the work in general may be stressful. Although working in a team can at times provide great support, group work can also be a source of stress if members do not do their part, conflicts develop, or communication is strained.

Resilience is a key component of being able to live a stable, satisfying, and productive life while coping with stresses and crises (Meyer, 2015). Resiliency can help people endure difficult times, bounce back, and maintain hope for the future (Muratori & Haynes, 2020). What makes one person more resilient than another? Although some people are naturally more resilient than others, resiliency can be learned or developed. Resilience is less about who a person is and more about how the person responds to a situation. Having confidence to handle a difficult situation, finding productive ways to respond to that situation, and using coping skills to successfully manage stressors will increase the likelihood of a positive outcome.

Many factors contribute to resilience, and some of the research on this topic was conducted with people who have endured disasters and traumas. Social support has been found to bolster resiliency in people who had endured two major natural disasters (Lee et al., 2019). Other studies have found that optimism, positive affect (e.g., happiness, excitement), and coping help protect against the development of mental disorders (Schaefer et al., 2018). Enhancing resiliency can lead to lower stress levels and increased positive well-being.

Being resilient typically helps a person cope better with stress and can decrease feelings of depression. Johnson et al. (2019) found that staff at universities (nonacademics) reported concerns about their working conditions, specifically increasing student numbers and related workload. Staff were troubled by pay and benefits, aspects of the job, and work relationships. Resilience is important early in the process of experiencing stressors because it influences how troublesome the presence of stressors is perceived (Johnson et al., 2019). These researchers concluded that employees with high levels of resilience may not perceive typical sources of stress as draining and are able to retain a more positive outlook.

Professional Competency Areas for Student Affairs Educators (ACPA–College Student Educators International & NASPA–Student Affairs Administrators in Higher Education, 2015) serves as a guide for higher education professionals and delineates essential knowledge, skills, and dispositions expected of all student affairs educators, regardless of functional area or specialization within the field. Resilience is addressed in this document, which recommends that higher education professionals "bolster [their] resiliency, including participating in stress-management activities, engaging in personal or spiritual exploration, and building healthier relationships inside and outside of the workplace" (p. 17). These suggestions include a number of recommendations that align with strategies that can help strengthen resilience. No one's life (or job) is without crises and disappointments; it is how you handle and view these setbacks that determines your outcome.

Personal Wellness and Self-Care

According to Corey et al. (2018), "Wellness is an individual's holistic approach to health over the life span" (p. 5), while self-care is an individual's specific attempts to improve their health to meet the challenges of the job. To achieve wellness, a person must be committed to achieving personal goals and making decisions that help them experience happiness and peace. The importance of personal wellness is understood to be a professional imperative. This is exemplified in ACPA and NASPA's (2015) *Professional Competency Areas for Student Affairs Educators*. The Personal and Ethical Foundations competency area (ACPA & NASPA, 2015) emphasizes, among other actions, a commitment to one's own wellness. It encourages higher education professionals to "articulate an understanding that wellness is a broad concept comprised of emotional, physical, social, environmental, relational, spiritual, moral, and intellectual elements" (p. 16).

One of the first modern wellness models was proposed by Bill Hettler (1976). These six domains include occupational, physical, social, intellectual, emotional, and spiritual. Over time, other wellness experts have expanded on the domains. Ohrt et al. (2019) recommended looking across these domains to identify declining wellness. Mind wellness could be impaired by being distracted at work and having a hard time concentrating when others are talking. A decrease in body wellness may manifest itself as sleep impairment and unpleasant feelings as one approaches their worksite. Signs that one's spiritual wellness is affected may include losing a sense of direction and purpose in one's life and neglecting spiritual or religious practices. A lack of empathy or an inability to connect with others can signal a decrease in emotional wellness. When a professional experiences conflictual communication with coworkers, students, or supervisors or interpersonal difficulties there may be a breakdown in their connection wellness. Make time to assess yourself across these domains and address these wellness deficits as they appear (Ohrt et al., 2019).

Self-care is one way to ensure personal wellness. Corey et al. (2018) defined *self-care* as specific attempts to improve one's own health to better meet the many challenges one faces. The authors warned that not engaging in self-care practices will leave one without the requisite energy or stamina to be present with others, which is a necessary condition for higher education professionals. In this field, self-care is an important topic to address and encourage. As stated earlier, higher education professionals are often charged to work long and unpredictable hours and to fulfill multiple roles simultaneously (Daut, 2016). Their concern for student well-being can be emotionally draining and demanding, which only serves to emphasize why they need to find time for their own self-care. As professionals in the field of higher education endure their work in helping roles, providing attention and care for students, they should also prioritize their own care (Daut, 2016). Taking care of others first requires self-care. The saying, "You need to fill your own bucket before you can fill others" is a good reminder to help ground and guide us.

One way to ensure self-care is to make time for yourself outside of work. What are you passionate about? What gives you fulfillment and joy? The answers to these questions will vary for each person. For some, spending time in body work (e.g., massage, yoga, stretching, exercise) brings great satisfaction and related health benefits. Exercise increases energy and may decrease mental fatigue. Many people find solace in spiritual practices, such as formal religion, meditation, and prayer. Spiritual practices can increase your sense of calmness, help you cope with stress, and increase your feeling of gratitude. Hobbies can also provide self-care. Hobbies can give you a break from work, induce feelings of purpose, and offer new challenges and experiences. Last, connecting with others in a group or social club is a great way to increase your network of support and find common interests with others.

Learning to balance work and leisure can be difficult. The term *work–life balance* may have different meanings for everyone. In this fast-paced technological society, it can be hard to disconnect from work. Smartphones provide a constant feed of texts and emails and ensure accessibility 24 hours a day, which can impinge on out-of-work recovery time and make it difficult to leave work at the office. However, stepping away and finding time apart from work is important. In most cases, the work will still be there when you are ready to face it again.

Finding a balance between work and life is essential to ensure you have time in your life for friends, family, and outside pursuits. The old proverb "All work and no play makes Jack a dull boy" still holds true. Be sure to take advantage of your vacation or leave time. Studies have shown that too many Americans do not utilize their vacation time (Sampson, 2019) and instead continue to work without a break. Those who do take vacations often check in with their jobs while they are away. To maintain a work–life balance, you may need to assert yourself at work, learn to say "no" at times, and set limits with your work colleagues.

If you're thinking about beginning to explore personal wellness and self-care, you may find free resources right on your campus. Most universities have fitness centers, yoga classes, and perhaps nature walks. If you feel you may need to talk to a professional, seeking services at the counseling center or from the employee assistance program on campus is a good place to start. Utilize your lunchtime break to step away from your desk, enjoy your meal outside, or take a brief walk around your building. Table 5.1 provides suggestions for many forms of self-care. The categories and recommended activities may overlap because some tasks will work in several domains.

It may take time to achieve a work–life balance and find self-care strategies that work for you. The activity you choose to do is not important, as long as you do something that you enjoy and recharges you. Ohrt et al. (2019) advised being mindful of which self-care activities are important to you and will be truly helpful. For example, if joining an exercise class is going to be stressful, choose something else. Commit to a wellness plan and find meaning not only in your work but also in your personal pursuits.

Table 5.1
Forms of Self-Care and Stress Reduction

Physical	Emotional	Social	Spiritual	Mental
Exercising	Talking with supportive friends and family	Taking a vacation	Meditating	Spending time by yourself
Eating a balanced diet	Expressing your emotions in a healthy way	Socializing	Attending religious services	Reading a book for pleasure
Doing tai chi	Engaging in counseling/therapy/self-growth	Visiting family	Praying	Learning something new
Practicing yoga	Playing with a pet	Spending time with friends	Developing a deeper sense of the universe	Watching a movie
Sleeping/napping	Engaging in positive self-talk	Nurturing relationships	Stating positive affirmations	Doing a puzzle or sudoku
Taking medication as prescribed	Practicing forgiveness	Saying "no" and setting healthy boundaries	Finding meaning in life	Listening to music
Attending medical appointments	Laughing		Repeating a mantra	Practicing deep breathing
Doing stretching exercises				Engaging in creative arts

Conclusion

Working in higher education can be exciting and rewarding. Spending time with students who are eager to learn and embark on a new phase of their life can bring the higher education professional joy. However, some aspects of work can be demanding and draining. Long work hours, taking work home, and the endless flood of emails and texts may leave some professionals feeling stressed. Recognizing the signs of stress and ensuring good self-care can help prevent more serious negative effects. Without time for hobbies, friends, and family, the higher education professional may suffer from burnout.

These feelings of hopelessness can impact the professional's work and attitude. Proper nutrition, sleep, and engaging regularly in pleasurable activities are critical to a healthy work–life balance.

References

ACPA–College Student Educators International & NASPA–Student Affairs Administrators in Higher Education. (2015). *Professional competency areas for student affairs educators.* https://www.naspa.org/images/uploads/main/ACPA_NASPA_Professional_Competencies_FINAL.pdf

American Psychological Association. (2017). *Stress in America: Coping with change.* https://www.apa.org/news/press/releases/stress/2017/technology-social-media.pdf

Barkhuizen, N., Rothmann, S., & Van de Vijver, F. J. (2014). Burnout and work engagement of academics in higher education institutions: Effects of dispositional optimism. *Stress and Health, 30*(4), 322–332. https://doi.org/10.1002/smi.2520

Barlow, D. H., Durand, V. M., & Hofmann, S. G. (2018). *Abnormal psychology: An integrative approach* (8th ed.). Cengage Learning.

Cohen, S., & Janicki-Devartis, D. (2009). Can we improve our physical health by altering our social networks? *Perspectives on Psychological Science, 4*(4), 375–378. https://doi.org/10.1111%2Fj.1745-6924.2009.01141.x

Corey, G., Corey, M. S., & Corey, C. (2019). *Issues and ethics in the helping profession* (10th ed.). Cengage Learning.

Corey, G., Muratori, M., Austin, J. T., & Austin, J. A. (2018). *Counselor self-care.* John Wiley & Sons.

Corey, M. S., & Corey, G. (2021). *Becoming a helper* (8th ed.). Cengage Learning.

Daut, C. (2016). A case for more yoga on campus: Yoga as self-care for higher education and student affairs professionals. *The Vermont Connection, 37*(6), 48–60. https://scholarworks.uvm.edu/tvc/vol37/iss1/6

DuBois, A. L., & Mistretta, M. A. (2020). *Overcoming burnout and compassion fatigue in schools: A guide for counselors, administrators, and educators.* Routledge.

Freudenberger, H. J. (1974). Staff burn-out. *Journal of Social Issues, 30*(1), 159–165. http://dx.doi.org/10.1111/j.1540-4560.1974.tb00706.x

Hakanen, J. J., & Schaufeli, W. B. (2012). Do burnout and work engagement predict depressive symptoms and life satisfaction? A three-wave 7-year prospective study. *Journal of Affective Disorders, 141*(2–3), 415–424. https://doi.org/10.1016/j.jad.2012.02.043

Hettler, B. (1976). *The six dimensions of wellness model.* https://www.heartcenteredpsychology.com/resources/2018/8/3/the-six-dimensions-of-wellness-model-by-dr-bill-hettler

Johnson, S. J., Willis, S. M., & Evans, J. (2019). An examination of stressors, strain, and resilience in academic and non-academic U.K. university job roles. *International Journal of Stress Management, 26*(2), 162. https://psycnet.apa.org/doi/10.1037/str0000096

Lee, J., Blackmon, B. J., Lee, J. Y., Cochran, D. M., Jr., & Rehner, T. A. (2019). An exploration of posttraumatic growth, loneliness, depression, resilience, and social capital among survivors of Hurricane Katrina and the Deepwater Horizon Oil Spill. *Journal of Community Psychology, 47*(2), 356–370. https://doi.org/10.1002/jcop.22125

Leiter, M. P., & Maslach, C. (2008). Early predictors of job burnout and engagement. *Journal of Applied Psychology, 93*(3), 498–512. https://doi.org/10.1037/0021-9010.93.3.498

MacKay, J. (2020, January 29). How to deal with burnout: Signs, symptoms, and strategies for getting you back on track after burning out. *RescueTime.* https://blog.rescuetime.com/burnout-syndrome-recovery

Maslach, C. (2003). *Burnout: The cost of caring.* Malor Books.

Maslach, C., & Leiter, M. P. (2016). Understanding the burnout experience: Recent research and its implications for psychiatry. *World Psychiatry, 15*(2), 103–111. https://doi.org/10.1002/wps.20311

Meyer, I. H. (2015). Resilience in the study of minority stress and health of sexual and gender minorities. *Psychology of Sexual Orientation and Gender Diversity, 2*(3), 209–213. https://doi.org/10.1037/sgd0000132

Muratori, M., & Haynes, R. H. (2020). *Coping skills for a stressful world: A workbook for counselors and clients.* John Wiley & Sons.

Ohrt, J. H., Clarke, P. B., & Conley, A. H. (2019). *Wellness counseling: A holistic approach to prevention and intervention.* John Wiley & Sons.

Poulsen, A. A., Meredith, P., Khan, A., Henderson, J., Castrisos, V., & Khan, S. R. (2014). Burnout and work engagement in occupational therapists. *British Journal of Occupational Therapy, 77*(3), 156–164. https://doi.org/10.4276%2F030802214X13941036266621

Pryce, J. G., Shackelford, K. K., & Pryce, D. H. (2007). *Secondary traumatic stress and the child welfare professional.* Lyceum Books.

Robertson, I., & Cooper, C. L. (2013). Resilience [Editorial]. *Stress and Health: Journal of the International Society for the Investigation of Stress, 29*(3), 175–176. https://doi.org/10.1002/smi.2512

Sampson, H. (2019, August 28). What does America have against vacation? *The Washington Post.* https://www.washingtonpost.com/travel/2019/08/28/what-does-america-have-against-vacation

Schaefer, L. M., Howell, K. H., Schwartz, L. E., Bottomley, J. S., & Crossnine, C. B. (2018). A concurrent examination of protective factors associated with resilience and posttraumatic growth following childhood victimization. *Child Abuse & Neglect, 85,* 17–27. https://doi.org/10.1016/j.chiabu.2018.08.019

Schueller, S. M., & Parks, A. C. (2014). The science of self-help: Translating positive psychology research into increased individual happiness. *European Psychologist, 19*(2), 145–155. https://doi.org/10.1027/1016-9040/a000181

Taylor, S. E. (2020). *Health Psychology* (11th ed.). McGraw-Hill Education.

Tull, A. (2006). Synergistic supervision, job satisfaction, and intention to turnover of new professionals in student affairs. *Journal of College Student Development, 47*(4), 465–480. https://doi.org/10.1353/csd.2006.0053

Werneburg, B. L., Jenkins, S. M., Friend, J. L., Berkland, B. E., Clark, M. M., Rosedahl, J. K., & Sood, A. (2018). Improving resiliency in healthcare employees. *American Journal of Health Behavior, 42*(1), 39–50. https://doi.org/10.5993/AJHB.42.1.4

CHAPTER 6

Cultural and Diversity Awareness

As student demographics at colleges and universities throughout the United States continue to shift, higher education professionals need to develop cultural understanding when helping students. According to the National Center for Education Statistics (n.d.), the overall college enrollment rate for traditional-aged students attending college between 2017 and 2028 projects a marked shift in demographics. The number of White students will decrease by 6%, the number of Black students will increase by 8%, and the number of Hispanic students will increase by 14%. There will also be a slight increase in Asian/Pacific Islander students, and a decrease in Native American/Alaska Native students (see Table 6.1). Colleges and universities will continue to become more and more diverse.

This chapter focuses on the cultural aspect of mental health and how it can impact the ways professionals support students in crisis. Many students face issues at home, struggle with stigma, and have other culturally based challenges surrounding mental health. In addition, for some students, the acculturation process is exacerbated by the stress of academic studies and university life. Race, gender, sexual identity, and other cultural aspects of identity, and the intersectionality of these identities, can all affect a student's mental health and the ability to succeed in college. This chapter will discuss those factors as well as how to create a culturally sensitive and supportive environment.

Table 6.1
Higher Education Enrollment by Race/Ethnicity

Between 2017 and 2028, enrollment of U.S. residents is projected to
↓ decrease 6% for students who are White (10.5 million vs. 9.9 million)
↑ increase 8% for students who are Black (2.5 million vs. 2.7 million)
↑ increase 14% for students who are Hispanic (3.5 million vs. 4.0 million)
↑ increase 2% for students who are Asian/Pacific Islander (1.3 million vs. 1.4 million)
↓ decrease 9% for students who are American Indian/Alaska Native (138,000 vs. 125,000)
↑ increase 1% for students who are of two or more races (700,000 vs. 705,000)

Note. Adapted from *Projections of Education Statistics to 2028,* by the National Center for Education Statistics, U.S. Department of Education, n.d. (https://nces.ed.gov/programs/PES/section-5.asp#7). In the public domain.

Current Climate

The events in spring 2020, historically marked by the killings of George Floyd, Breonna Taylor, and others, sparked a new era on college campuses. With the Black Lives Matter movement, the climate on campuses radically shifted. College and university leaders across the country began issuing statements to their students and alumni that they supported their Black students and were committed to addressing issues of racism on campus and in the classroom. But, in a departure from similar events in the past, students began demanding more action, not just words and letters. It became apparent that it was time for institutional leadership to take a hard look at their curriculum, teaching, and hiring practices. While these actions are instrumental in making fundamental change, colleges and universities cannot ignore the mental distress being placed on their Black, Indigenous, and People of Color (BIPOC) students. Taking important steps to improve the emotional health of BIPOC students is an important step in creating an inclusive and positive learning environment for all students.

Along with the racial inequities being brought to the forefront, other underserved populations have continued to come to campuses needing the full support and assistance of the administration, faculty, and their peers. Students with disabilities, those who identify with the LGBTQIA+ community, and other underrepresented students have increased access to campuses across the country. With this access comes the added responsibility for institutions to provide an environment that supports these students' educational and emotional needs.

BIPOC Students

All students experience some level of stress, not only as they transition to college but throughout their journey as college students. For underrespresented students, however, this stress is exacerbated. Many report experiencing "imposter syndrome" where they do not truly feel they deserve to be there (Cokley et al., 2013). The imposter phenomenon has been tied to clinically significant mental health symptoms of depression, generalized anxiety, and low self-esteem (Chrisman et al., 1995; MacGeorge et al., 2008). Higher education professionals must be aware of these symptoms and conditions when working with students.

In addition to the typical pressures of college life, these students must deal with the additional stressors of racism, discrimination, difficulties trying to fit in, insensitive comments from peers and others, and other aspects of being from an underrepresented population (Cokley et al, 2013; Goodman & West-Olatunji, 2010; Okazaki, 2009). These experiences can occur in and out of the classroom and may result from subtle or overtly racist educational policies, professors who are culturally insensitive in their teaching and curricular design, and interracial group tension (Chiu & Ring, 1998). Racial and ethnic minority students often seek mental health treatment at lower rates than their White peers (Miranda et al., 2015). They report more barriers, such as financial concerns and time constraints, and suffer more highly from the stigma related to seeking help. These issues, coupled with negative stereotypes and cultural inconsistencies, can put underrepresented students at increased risk for mental health concerns.

These factors have contributed to the development of what is referred to as "minority status stress," often forcing these students to adapt their own coping mechanisms (Greer & Brown, 2011). This process can sometimes lead to a more difficult adjustment to college and eventual feelings of depression and loneliness. Coupled with imposter syndrome, this added stress can cause underrepresented students to have increased mental health issues.

The most common reasons that these students avoid help-seeking are that they prefer to handle their problems on their own, they think their stress or concerns are normal and do not require support, they are getting help from other sources, and they lack the time (Miranda et al., 2015). Stigma is a far greater concern among racial/ethnic minorities than White students (Miranda et al., 2015). Within many racial and ethnic minority cultures, help-seeking causes a fear of looking crazy or weak. These students do not often see role models in their cultures speaking openly about struggling with mental health. Families often prefer to keep such issues private and do not want to involve others. Additionally, some students prefer to seek alternative methods to help them with their struggles: Seeking support from avenues such as family, friends, religious guides, herbalists, and others can sometimes be more culturally aligned.

LGBTQIA+ Students

LGBTQIA+ students are at high risk for mental health problems and suicidal behaviors, and the rate of suicide attempts is greater among this population compared to their peers (Bouris & Hill, 2017; D'Augelli et al., 2001; Su et al., 2016). Similar to BIPOC students who have the added stress of their minority status, LGBTQIA+ students are dealing with the normal stressors of adolescence combined with the added pressures of understanding and then disclosing their sexual identity to family and friends (Bouris & Hill, 2017; Brown et al., 2004). These students deal with the pressures of having their sexual identity discovered, disclosing their sexual orientation, and being ridiculed by others. They sometimes find themselves on campuses that are neither supportive nor inclusive of their identities, and they might struggle to find supportive services. Many students in the LGBTQIA+ community often experience victimization, discrimination, and marginalization (Bochenek & Brown, 2001; Kosciw et al., 2010). For BIPOC LBGTQIA+ students, these problems can be exacerbated by further issues of racism and discrimination. While these issues are concerning and need to be addressed for their impact on students' overall well-being, they can also affect these students' success in the classroom (Murdock & Bolch, 2005; Russell et al., 2001). When faculty and staff take proactive steps to create a safe and welcoming environment, they can help undo the negative effects LGBTQIA+ students have experienced from years of feeling marginalized and persecuted (Bochenek & Brown, 2001; Russell et al., 2001). When LGBTQIA+ students are able to find and connect with supportive faculty and staff, they show improvement in their overall mental health (Goodenow et al., 2006) and academic performance (Russell et al., 2001).

Students With Disabilities

Since the Americans With Disabilities Act of 1990, access to higher education for students with disabilities has continued to increase. Institutions have a legal obligation to provide reasonable accommodations—both in and outside of the classroom—to any and all students who self-disclose a need. As the population of students with disabilities on campus grows, higher education professionals must understand and be sensitive to the different needs of this population.

Like BIPOC and LGBTQIA+ students, students with disabilities face similar challenges when starting their college journey. Not only do they have the typical transitional issues, but they have the additional layer of navigating their disabilities, managing their accommodations, and facing obstacles unique to their circumstances (Shepler & Woosley, 2012). Not every disability is the same or manifests itself in the same manner for every student. Like other underrepresented populations, students with disabilities or impairments suffer from discrimination, stigmatization, and lack of inclusion. Students with disabilities often feel less comfortable in their classes and with their faculty, and they have experienced higher levels of discrimination than their nondisabled peers (Aquino et al., 2017; Evans et al., 2017). This issue is increased even further for BIPOC and LGBTQIA+ students. Taking care to provide an inclusive environment is an important step in creating a positive college experience and facilitating students' educational and development success (Pascarella & Terenzini, 2005; Reason & Rankin, 2006; Tinto, 1993).

Some of the ways higher education professionals can support students with disabilities is simply by being aware of how to be helpful and sensitive to the barriers and challenges these students may be facing. When working with visually impaired students, take care not to grab for them or offer them an elbow—they have developed their own abilities to navigate independently. Help them orient themselves to where they are physically and assist with technology access. With hearing-impaired students, some people have a tendency to raise their voice, thinking this will help the student understand them. This is a common misconception and typically not helpful. The best way to assist these students is to speak clearly and with a level tone, and to maintain eye contact. When working with students on the autism spectrum, it is best to give direct, explicit, and concrete directions. These students often will not pick up on nonverbal cues, so being very clear in what is expected will serve them well. It is also important to keep in mind challenges of the physical campus: Is a class being taught in a room that might be difficult for a student with mobility issues to navigate? Sometimes professors change classrooms at the last minute; they should be mindful of how the change might impact their students. Also consider programming spaces—are they accessible to all students? How is the campus maintained after certain weather events? Are sidewalks quickly cleared of snow, ice, or other debris? Lastly, when working with students with disabilities, always remember to use person-first language; students are not defined by their disabilities—say "the student who is visually impaired," not "the blind student." Taking care to use inclusive language will go a long way to creating a welcoming and supportive environment.

Students with disabilities are often less likely to feel engaged in their community or may need help with self-advocacy and efficacy (Shepler & Woosley, 2012). Higher education professionals can help these students feel connected and included in campus life by encouraging them to join clubs and organizations, taking an active role in their academic planning, and increasing their levels of self-advocacy and independence. Campuses can also increase student success by offering programming aimed at students with disabilities, assigning faculty and staff mentors, and creating student organizations for students with disabilities.

What Can Be Done?

Campus diversity and acceptance of underrepresented populations has certainly increased, but these students continue to face discrimination and stigma. One of the main ways higher education professionals can help underrepresented students succeed in college and feel more included is to ensure they have the support and services they need. That means hiring clinicians for counseling centers who represent these students in numbers that are reflective of the population—not just one or two. BIPOC students are less likely to seek help from the counseling center due to mistrust of White counselors whom they perceive as not having adequate cultural understanding to provide them with the assistance they need (Miranda et al., 2015). These students need to know they can find a counselor who shares their lived experiences. Counseling centers need to take care to offer programming that is reflective of and appeals to a culturally diverse student body. For example, many programs focus on empathy and listening. There is a cultural element that needs to be understood and recongnized when discussing communication techniques. It is important to recognize cultural influences as well surrounding counseling when creating programs with the goal of reducing stigma. Some strategies that are more impactful than traditional programming include social media interventions, campuswide opt-out mental health checkups, and partnerships with local organizations that support underserved communities. This same philosophy applies to higher education staff. Institutions need to hire BIPOC higher education professionals, members of the LGBTQIA+ community, and those with disabilities in a manner more reflective of the student demographic population.

Training and Professional Development

The higher education professionals who are in the best positions to help underrepresented students often lack the understanding needed to work with these populations without further alienating, stigmatizing, or stereotyping them (Hong, 2015; Hurtado & Guillermo-Wann, 2013; Thompson, 2014). Higher education professionals need training on the various development theories and practices to allow them to practice empathy and understanding when talking with students about personal issues (Stewart, 2020). This training would also allow higher education professionals to more easily encourage mental health counseling. There are institutes such as the YES Institute in South Florida whose mission is to address the root causes of discrimination, harassment, and suicide through education, training, and dialogue around issues of gender and orientation. Partnering with an organization similar to the YES Institute would be a positive step toward opening up discussion and creating an inclusive and welcoming environment for all students.

As issues of bias and discrimination continue on campus, a key strategy to combat the problem is increased professional development for faculty and staff. This can have a significant impact on changing beliefs held by faculty and staff and empowering higher education professionals to encourage intervention (Greytak et al., 2013). The more professionals stay educated about the issues facing their students, the better equipped they will be to create supportive and inclusive communities (Greytak et al., 2013). Training also fosters empathy and understanding within higher education professionals and increases their confidence when handling issues that may have been beyond their comfort zone prior to training. It is important to create a campus climate that both encourages and increases access to the counseling center. This can be done by increasing awareness and training while decreasing stigma.

More recently, there have been calls within the field of higher education from faculty, staff, and students for the establishment of racial violence prevention offices and reporting systems. Modeled after Title IX offices, these offices would provide interventions and training as well as allow a channel for reporting and responding to racial violence on campus. Without such an office, BIPOC students often perceive that their needs and experiences are not as valued, and actions taken against them are not as important or serious.

Conclusion

Campuses should strive to create an environment where students feel respected and appreciated for what they bring to the community; this is an essential element of a campus culture committed to diversity and inclusion (Harbour & Greenberg, 2017). Institutions can create this environment by educating staff about systemic racism and other inequities within society and educational systems so that they are better equipped to support students. Unfortunately, there is no one type of training that will succeed on every campus. Each campus needs to take measures to determine what training and education will best match its own particular goals and needs (Carter, 2020).

Higher education professionals who work with underrepresented populations can focus on what unites students, rather than what divides them. Helping students advocate for themselves and engage in activism has been found to be a positive and productive coping mechanism (Szymanski, 2012). Encouraging students to redirect their energy into activism empowers those who may feel marginalized or discriminated against. Counseling centers can create student groups geared toward specific underrepresented populations, giving them a place to talk with others who might be experiencing similar issues. Higher education professionals can point students toward these resources and advocate for them. And it is essential professionals intervene when they witness acts of bullying or harassment. Educators are often inconsistent in calling out behaviors that are homophobic, transphobic, racist, and so on. This silence is damaging to the campus community and needs to be addressed through training and education. Higher education professionals are key stakeholders in helping students advocate for themselves.

References

Aquino, K. C., Alhaddab, T. A., & Kim, E. (2017). Does disability matter? Students' satisfaction with college experiences. In E. Kim & K. C. Aquino (Eds.), *Disability as diversity in higher education: Policies and practices to enhance student success* (pp. 47–60). Routledge.

Bochenek, M., & Brown, A. W. (2001). *Hatred in the hallways: Violence and discrimination against lesbian, gay, bisexual, and transgender students in U.S. schools*. Human Rights Watch.

Bouris, A., & Hill, B. (2017). Out on campus: Meeting the mental health needs of sexual and gender minority college students. *Journal of Adolescent Health, 61,* 271–272. https://doi.org/10.1016/j.jadohealth.2017.06.002

Brown, R. D., Clarke, B., Gortmaker, V., & Robinson-Keilig, R. (2004). Assessing the campus climate for gay, lesbian, bisexual, and transgender (GLBT) students using a multiple perspectives approach. *Journal of College Student Development, 45*(1), 8–26. https://doi.org/10.1353/csd.2004.0003

Carter, E. (2020, June 22). Restructure your organization to actually advance racial justice. *Harvard Business Review*. https://hbr.org/2020/06/restructure-your-organization-to-actually-advance-racial-justice

Chiu, Y.-W., & Ring, J. M. (1998). Chinese and Vietnamese immigrant adolescents under pressure: Identifying stressors and interventions. *Professional Psychology: Research and Practice, 29*(5), 444–449. https://doi.org/10.1037/0735-7028.29.5.444

Chrisman, S. M., Pieper, W. A., Clance, P. R., Holland, C. L., & Glickauf-Hughes, C. (1995). Validation of the clance imposter phenomenon scale. *Journal of Personality Assessment, 65*(3), 456–467. https://doi.org/10.1207/s15327752jpa6503_6

Cokley, K, McClain, S., Enciso, A., & Martinez, M. (2013). An examination of the impact of minority status stress and impostor feelings on the mental health of diverse ethnic minority college students. *Journal of Multicultural Counseling and Development, 41*(2), 82–95. https://doi.org/10.1002/j.2161-1912.2013.00029.x

D'Augelli, A. R., Hershberger, S. L., & Pilkington, N. W. (2001). Suicidality patterns and sexual orientation-related factors among lesbian, gay, and bisexual youths. *Suicide and Life Threatening Behavior, 31*(3), 250–265. https://doi.org/10.1521/suli.31.3.250.24246

Evans, N. J., Broido, E. M., Brown, K. R., & Wilke, A. K. (2017). *Disability in higher education: A social justice approach*. Jossey-Bass.

Goodenow, C., Szalacha, L., & Westheimer, K. (2006). School support groups, other school factors, and the safety of sexual minority adolescents. *Psychology in the Schools, 43*(5), 573–589. https://doi.org/10.1002/pits.20173

Goodman, R. D., & West-Olatunji, C. A. (2010). Educational hegemony, traumatic stress, and African American and Latino American students. *Journal of Multicultural Counseling and Development, 38*(3), 176–186. https://doi.org/10.1002/j.2161-1912.2010.tb00125.x

Greer, T. M., & Brown, P. (2011). Minority status stress and coping processes among African American college students. *Journal of Diversity in Higher Education, 4*(1), 26–38. https://doi.org/10.1037/a0021267

Greytak, E. A., Kosciw, J. G., & Boesen, M. J. (2013). Educating the educator: Creating supportive school personnel through professional development. *Journal of School Violence, 12*(1), 80–97. https://doi.org/10.1080/15388220.2012.731586

Harbour, W., & Greenberg, D. (2017). *NCCSD research brief: Campus climate and students with disabilities* (Vol. 1, No. 2). National Center for College Students with Disabilities.

Hong, B. S. S. (2015). Qualitative analysis of the barriers college students with disabilities experience in higher education. *Journal of College Student Development, 56*(3), 209–226. https://doi.org/10.1353/csd.2015.0032

Hurtado, S., & Guillermo-Wann, C. (2013). *Diverse learning environments: Assessing and creating conditions for student success—Final report to the Ford Foundation.* Higher Education Research Institute, University of California, Los Angeles. https://www.heri.ucla.edu/ford/DiverseLearningEnvironments.pdf

Kosciw, J., Greytak, E., Diaz, E., & Barkiewicz, M. J. (2010). *The 2009 national school climate survey: The experiences of lesbian, gay, bisexual, and transgender youth in our nation's schools.* Gay, Lesbian and Straight Education Network.

MacGeorge, E. L., Feng, B., & Thompson, E. R. (2008). "Good" and "bad" advice: How to advise more effectively. In M. Motley (Ed.), *Applied interpersonal communication: Behaviors that affect outcomes* (pp. 145–164). Sage.

Miranda, R., Soffer, A., Polanco-Roman, L., Wheeler, A., & Moore, A. (2015). Mental health treatment barriers among racial/ethnic minority versus white young adults 6 months after intake at a college counseling center. *Journal of American College Health, 63*(5), 291–298. https://doi.org/10.1080/07448481.2015.1015024

Murdock, T. B., & Bolch, M. B. (2005). Risk and protective factors for poor school adjustment in lesbian, gay, and bisexual (LGB) high school youth: Variable and person-centered analyses. *Psychology in the Schools, 42*(2), 159–172. https://doi.org/10.1002/pits.20054

National Center for Education Statistics. (n.d.). *Projections of eduction statistics to 2028.* https://nces.ed.gov/programs/PES/section-5.asp#7

Okazaki, S. (2009). Impact of racism on ethnic minority mental health. *Perspectives on Psychological Science, 4*(1), 103–107. https://doi.org/10.1111/j.1745-6924.2009.01099.x

Pascarella, E., & Terenzini, P. T. (2005). *How college affects students: A third decade of research* (Vol. 2). Jossey-Bass.

Reason, R. D., & Rankin, S. R. (2006). College students' experiences and perceptions of harassment on campus: An exploration of gender differences. *College Student Affairs Journal, 26*(1), 7–29.

Russell, S. T., Seif, H., & Truong, N. L. (2001). School outcomes of sexual minority youth in the United States: Evidence from a national study. *Journal of Adolescence, 24*(1), 111–127. https://doi.org/10.1006/jado.2000.0365

Shepler, D., & Woosley, S. (2012). Understanding the early integration experiences of college students with disabilities. *Journal of Postsecondary Education and Disability, 25*(1), 37–50.

Stewart, J. F., Mallery, C., & Choi, J. (2013). College student persistence: A multilevel analysis of distance learning course completion at the crossroads of disability status. *Journal of College Student Retention, 15*(3), 367–385. https://doi.org/10.2190/CS.15.3.d

Su, D., Irwin, J., Fisher, C., Ramos, A., Kelley, M., Mendoza, D., & Coleman, J. (2016). Mental health disparities within the LGBT population: A comparison between transgender and nontransgender individuals. *Transgender Health, 1*(1), 12–20. https://doi.org/10.1089/trgh.2015.0001

Szymanski, D. M. (2012). Racist events and individual coping styles as predictors of African American activism. *Journal of Black Psychology, 38*(3), 342–367. https://doi.org/10.1177/0095798411424744

Thompson, T. L. (2014). Postsecondary education for people with intellectual disabilities. In M. L. Vance, N. E. Lipsitz, & K. Parks (Eds.), *Beyond the Americans with Disabilities Act: Inclusive policy and practice for higher education* (pp. 97–110). NASPA–Student Affairs Administrators in Higher Education.

Tinto, V. (1993). *Leaving college: Rethinking the causes and cures of student attrition* (2nd ed.). University of Chicago Press.

CHAPTER 7

Anxiety and Stress

The adjustment to college life can contribute to feelings of anxiety and stress in students. Such stress can manifest itself in a variety of ways such as somatic concerns, difficulty concentrating, or headaches. College seniors may fear what awaits them after college, and the pressure to gain employment or pursue graduate studies may feel daunting. This chapter will discuss signs and symptoms of anxiety and stress, allowing the higher education professional to identify them in students and make appropriate recommendations. Learning to recognize and manage stress in students is one way in which higher education professionals can assist them.

Basic Signs and Symptoms of Anxiety and Stress

The demands of college life, living away from home, navigating roommates, and managing multiple responsibilities can result in anxiety and stress for some students. Although feelings of stress are expected with the intense workload associated with college, some students may enter campus with preexisting anxiety disorders that worsen under these conditions. College also involves a huge developmental progression for students as they become adults; for many freshmen, it is their first experience with independence and no parental monitoring or scheduling (Aaron et al., 2011). As students prepare to graduate—and think about leaving the comfort of college life—they may feel overwhelming anxiety about what comes next.

Anxiety is relatively common among college students, who are facing a wide range of new and demanding responsibilities. Anxiety disorders are the most commonly diagnosed and treated mental health conditions on college campuses today, according to the 2022 American College Health Association (ACHA) National College Health Assessment. The study found that in fall 2021, almost 30% of college students reported having anxiety to the extent that it affected their academic performance.

Case Study

Soledad wanted to go to a "good college." Both of her parents had advanced degrees, and she knew she was expected to go to college and graduate school. When she got into an elite private college on a tennis scholarship, she was thrilled. She had practiced for years at her sport, taking lessons, being part of travel teams, and missing out on a lot of school socialization due to her commitment to the sport. School work came fairly easy to her, but balancing academics and athletics had been challenging in her last 2 years of high school. When she arrived at her prestigious college, she was not prepared for how smart everyone else was. It seemed like everyone was the valedictorian at their school and all her teammates were great players, often having won their state championships. Soledad had to study for many hours at the library and still felt like she did not have enough time to get all her work done.

> She was fighting for her position on the team, and her coach had her playing at a lower position than she was used to. After practice, she was exhausted but had to study to keep her grades up. Before tests, she would experience intense anxiety at the thought that she might fail and thus lose her scholarship. Pain in her stomach was common and sometimes she had trouble eating.

There are many categories of anxiety. Some people feel anxious all the time about everything. They worry about both small details and big events. Typically, they will have a concern about something specific (e.g., getting the position they applied for in the lab), but once that event passes, their anxiety will find a new focus. This condition is what mental health experts call *generalized anxiety disorder*. It usually manifests itself in irritability, muscle tension, trouble sleeping, and feeling "on edge." Students with generalized anxiety disorder likely experienced it before they came to college; however, the condition may intensify once they settle into college life. Psychosomatic symptoms including headaches or stomach distress tend to be more common displays of anxiety among underrepresented populations (Ratanasiripong et al., 2012). Soledad's pain in her stomach, which kept her from eating, is likely an example of a psychosomatic symptom. So, these students may not report feelings of anxiety directly. For other students, their anxiety is tied to a specific place or situation; this can be called a *phobia*. Some phobias include fear of animals, thunder, needles, or crowded areas. For students with phobias, anxiety is displayed only if they must encounter or think about encountering the feared object. For example, a student who is afraid of dogs and just found out her sorority is hosting an event at a pet shelter may have anticipatory anxiety about the upcoming event and try at all costs not to attend.

> **Case Study**
>
> Elijiah had declared pre-med as his major. He was currently taking organic chemistry, biology, and physiology, and working at a lab on campus. He was really struggling with biology and often spent hours reading the book and reviewing the recorded lectures. One night in the library, he felt a bit dizzy, his palms were sweaty, and his heart was pounding. He was convinced he was having a heart attack. His friend took him to the campus health center, where he was examined by a physician. At the end of the exam, the physician told Elijah that he was having a panic attack. The physician suggested Elijah find ways to manage his anxiety and referred him to the campus counseling center.

Elijah was experiencing another type of anxiety: *panic attacks*. They are intense feelings of anxiety that can cause an increased heart rate, sweating, trembling or shaking, and dizziness. Panic attacks typically last only a few minutes, but the person who has them may worry about having more in the future. Because panic attacks are very physical in nature, they are often confused with heart attacks. *Social anxiety,* another anxiety disorder, manifests as an intense fear or anxiety about social situations; the individual is mainly concerned about possibly being scrutinized by others. Such situations can include chatting with others, eating in front of others, or having to give a speech. It is easy to see that these social circumstances can occur almost daily during college life and cause the student extreme anxiety. Students with social anxiety fear that they will be humiliated or embarrassed in these social settings and so avoid them entirely or endure them with anxiety. The ACHA (2022) study showed that 76% of college students sought treatment for anxiety disorders including panic attacks, generalized anxiety disorder, and social disorder within the last 12 months. The most commonly reported treatment for these students (44%) was medication and therapy. These conditions impact students' ability to function, as 28% reported their condition delayed their graduation and 29% reported an impact on their classwork.

There are several other sources of anxiety for students. Sprung and Rogers (2020) reported that career indecision is a common trigger of anxiety among college students. Although some students come to campus with an intended major and projected career choice, many are unsure of what they want to study or how they want to spend the rest of their lives. Pressure to declare a major, and thus a subsequent career, can provoke anxiety. Some students must work throughout college, whether it be as residence hall assistants, as teaching assistants, or in off-campus jobs. In fact, some studies show that students are increasingly likely to work while in college. Roughly 43% of undergraduate students are employed full time, and 81% are employed part time (National Center for Education Statistics, 2019). Students who work may feel worried about finances and paying for college. Those students who have less of a work–life balance are likely to report increased anxiety and symptoms of depression (Sprung & Rogers, 2020). Work–life balance is also strongly correlated with perceived stress. When students cannot achieve work–life balance, it contributes to their feelings of anxiety and depression. Transfer students have also been found to have high rates of anxiety (Cheung et al., 2020). These students are often experiencing a double transition—the transition associated with a new stage of life added to the transition of adjusting to a new college.

Stress

Stress is a normal part of life; without stress, we would be unmotivated. As Bamber and Kraenzle Schneider (2016) stated, "Stress at low levels can be beneficial, motivating students to perform well and preserve their mental and physical well-being" (p. 1). However, stress can be problematic when experienced at high levels. In the ACHA (2022) study, 39% of students reported that stress negatively affected their academics. Students feel the most stress when their coping resources are taxed beyond their limits.

Students may worry about events that are going to occur in the future, such as an examination (anticipatory stress); others may have concerns about something that is happening currently (acute stress), such as feeling anxious while making a class presentation (Conley & Lehman, 2012). Repeated exposure to academic stress can potentially impact students' physical health. Stress can affect the immune system, and it can alter attention and concentration (Shankar & Park, 2016). Long-term exposure to stress and anxiety can cause physical problems, including heart disease.

Some students will report working better under stress ("I study the most right before an exam and do well") while others may be overwhelmed by stress and not able to rise to the demands ("I just can't study thinking about all I have to do, and I end up doing nothing"). College is a hectic time for all students as they adjust to new social and academic demands. It may be particularly stressful for international students who are adapting to a new culture and (often) studying in a non-native language.

College Parents of America (2019) reported on the five main causes of stress for college students: unhealthy competition about GPAs, parents' expectations and parenting style, homesickness, social anxiety, and financial burden. Some students experience all five, and some may experience only one—but that one may cause enough stress to interfere with their functioning.

Everyone experiences stress; it is how a person responds to it that determines whether it becomes problematic. Research is mixed in demonstrating that students under stress engage in unhealthy habits such as binge eating (or skipping meals), sedentary behavior, drinking, or smoking (see Pelletier et al., 2016). But it is clear that students need psychological resources—that is, skills, beliefs, and attitudes that are learned through life experience—to respond to stress (Galloway Burke et al., 2017). Some examples of psychological resources are having faith in a higher power, grit, adequate problem-solving strategies, and regular self-care. It is often the role of student affairs to offer educational programming that gives psychological resources to students who may come to campus without them. This effort could take the form of workshops on problem solving, stress management techniques (e.g., yoga, meditation), and instruction on how to draw support from peers.

Some college students who are away from home for the first time may experience *homesickness*. They may be living across the country from their family and support network and learning to adjust to many new things. But some feelings of homesickness have been found to be beneficial. Sun and Hagedorn (2016) discovered that college students who experienced mild symptoms of homesickness were motivated to develop personal coping skills and establish new and healthy relationships. For most students, there is an initial adjustment period, but as they make friends, begin to feel more comfortable on campus, get more involved, and develop their friendships, their feelings of homesickness wane (Watson & Faucher, 2020).

College relationships are another frequent source of stress. Research has identified romantic relationships as a concern that leads many college students to seek counseling (Price et al., 2016). Because many of these relationships are just forming in college, students may be intensely affected by the highs and lows they experience. While a partner can be a great source of support, some college relationships are damaged by infidelity and poor communication. Social media has also been found to affect students stress and anxiety levels. FOMO, or the fear of missing out, is often blamed for addictive social media usage, as people fear other people are having more fun (Moore & Craciun, 2020). Additionally, compulsive use of social media may result in cyberbullying, pressure to maintain updates, and stress over others' posts.

Test Anxiety

Thousands of college students are affected by test anxiety (Chappell et al., 2005; Spielberger et al., 2015). Testing is not new to students; however, the high stakes of college grades may add to the pressure students feel to perform well. Tests can affect both short-term and long-term goals for students. Many may worry about their GPAs and how grades may affect acceptance to graduate school. Writing papers, studying, and taking exams are sources of considerable stress (Hughes, 2004, 2005), and although some anxiety is good (it can motivate a student to study and prepare), too much anxiety may interfere with a student's ability to perform. In some cases, anxiety may peak during an examination to the extent that students may experience a racing heart, sweaty palms, and dry mouth. Research has found that those with test anxiety may engage in negative thoughts, including catastrophizing (Putwain et al., 2010). They may engage in self-statements such as, "I think I am going to fail." Students with test anxiety worry about their performance on tests and many ruminate before the exam. They may delay doing assignments. The concern about test anxiety among college students is that it puts them at a greater risk of poor academic performance and potential school dropout (Gerwing et al., 2015). Some groups, such as women and students with learning disabilities, may be more prone to test anxiety (Gerwing et al., 2015).

Approaching Anxiety With Students

The signs and symptoms of anxiety may be obvious to the higher education professional. Students may appear jittery and on edge, and they may report having difficulty concentrating. Because stress is a universally experienced condition, discussing it with the student will likely be accepted without protest or denial. Framing what you see as anxiety as stress is one approach: "You seem really stressed out lately. What's going on?" This open-ended inquiry may yield some more information. Essentially, you want to get to the point with students where you learn enough to determine if it is stress or anxiety and if resources or professional help is warranted.

When, in talking to the student, signs of anxiety are evident, use the encounter as an opportunity to approach the issue and gently point out what you notice—for example, "You seem to be really focused on this issue and can't let it go. Are you feeling anxious about it?" Some students with anxiety perform what we call "mental gymnastics," ruminating about an issue, talking nonstop about it, playing out every possible scenario in their mind, and clearly worrying about the outcome. Bringing this behavior to the student's attention is one way to create awareness: "This upcoming presentation has really got you going. You seem to be thinking a lot about it. Have you been able to get your other work done?" The reply to this question can help you determine how disruptive these feelings of stress or anxiety truly are.

> **Case Study**
>
> Jesse had a mandatory chemistry lab on Friday after class; however, this was the same time his fraternity was conducting a leadership training that he was expected to attend. He worried nonstop about what to do about the conflict. He had trouble sleeping and obsessed about the outcome of his dilemma. For days, it was all he could think about. Jesse ran through the scenario with anyone who would listen, trying to gain feedback and guidance. He often seemed on the verge of tears.

There are many ways the higher education professional can intervene with students who experience anxiety and stress. For example, Sprung and Rogers (2020) advised that simply educating working students about the concept of work–life balance and its inherent struggles can help them alter their perceptions about how to deal with conflicts. If students accept that life in college will be a balancing act, they will be better able to plan. Being organized about school and outside work, including having time management skills, can help decrease stress and anxiety. Some research has shown that stress management programs may be helpful for students with low levels of anxiety (Hirokawa et al., 2002). Training students on adaptive/active coping strategies such as cognitive reappraisal (e.g., thinking about the situation in other ways) and social skills may help with those who have low levels of anxiety. In the case of Jesse, helping him find a way to talk to both his chemistry professor and his fraternity about the conflict will move him toward a possible solution.

Bamber and Morpeth (2019) found that mind-based interventions had a large and significant effect in decreasing anxiety in undergraduate students. The most effective interventions have at least eight sessions; student affairs offices may want to offer such programming. Pelletier et al. (2016) recommended that campus health centers offer stress management groups and provide other resources to ease the burden of stress on students, particularly students of color, who are more likely to experience adverse health outcomes. Tools for meal planning and smoking cessation would also be helpful, as students may eat erratically and turn to smoking when stressed out.

Adequate exam preparation and good test-taking skills also typically help to combat feelings of anxiety in students. Higher education professionals can recommend that students be sufficiently prepared for a test, get a good night's sleep the night before, and eat before the exam. Some students must learn to create a study environment that is free from distractions, manage time appropriately, and relax by taking a few deep breaths before heading into exams. Because much of the stress experienced by college students relates to academics, Tripathi and Sharma (2013) suggested students take advantage of teacher resources (e.g., office hours), join a study group, begin assignments in advance to prepare for potential technology difficulties, and schedule "down time" to recharge. Carving out time to see friends and pursue hobbies is critical to reducing stress.

Mahmoud et al. (2012) in a study of 257 undergraduate students found that the students' anxiety was primarily related to negative thinking and maladaptive coping. The authors discovered that negative thinking predicts more frequent use of maladaptive coping strategies and higher levels of anxiety. Generally, students who used adaptive coping, positive thinking, religious involvement, and social support tended to have more life satisfaction; students who used maladaptive coping were those who lived alone, engaged in negative thinking, and had more anxiety. Higher education professionals can inquire about these areas—for example, "Maria, you sound very stressed out about classes and assignments. Do you ever find time to relax with friends and step away from school for a while?" or "Luke, I know you have told me about going to services before; are you able to find any time to practice spirituality or attend religious services on campus? Lots of people find that helps with managing stress."

Many suggested activities to help reduce student anxiety include art, journaling, exercise, music therapy, and, most recently, mindfulness-based exercises such as meditation. Bamber and Kraenzle Schneider (2016) noted that mindfulness-based interventions focus on increasing an individual's awareness of the present moment and bodily sensations, the mind–body connection, and attention; these exercises mainly underscore having nonjudgmental thoughts. Some specific interventions might be mindfulness meditation and diaphragmatic breathing, which help to bring awareness to unconscious thoughts, feelings, and behaviors. Web-based platforms that offer mindfulness-based training may be of interest to college students struggling with anxiety and stress. Eustis et al. (2018) created a brief three-session, web-based, therapist-assisted, acceptance-based behavioral intervention targeting anxiety for college students. The intervention, called Surviving and Thriving During Stress, included psychoeducation, mindfulness, and values exercises. The higher education professional should be aware of such resources (both on campus and online) for those students who may be struggling with low to moderate levels of anxiety and stress.

When and How to Make a Referral to Counseling

Students with anxiety or stress that is starting to affect their daily functioning or their physical health most likely need some type of professional intervention. Conditions that last only a few days, can be controlled with effort, and are limited to a specific issue can be considered healthy or "normal" (Watson & Faucher, 2020); however, stress and anxiety that is pervasive and uncontrollable is unhealthy. There are many indicators that a student should be referred to a mental health professional for unhealthy anxiety. These include if the student reports a previous history of anxiety, the anxiety is leading to insomnia, the student is experiencing panic attacks, or the anxiety seems to be accompanied by depression. Because anxiety can progress to the point of severe depression or potentially suicidal ideation, referral to a professional is key. The higher education professional should ask students whether they have ever experienced these symptoms or issues before. As stated earlier, many students may come to campus with preexisitng anxiety disorders. Finding out if a student had professional help before arriving on campus may make it easier to suggest that now is another time when the student could find such intervention helpful.

The best way to approach professional intervention with students is to help them see the negative effects of stress or anxiety on them. "Latoya, each time we speak, you seem to be more and more worried about your classes and grades. I can see how this worry seems to affect your mood. Do you think you might want to try to work on ways to manage it?" This type of statement acknowledges the student's anxiety but gives the student the choice to accept help or not. The next step would be to recommend seeking help from the campus counseling center. This referral can be made by saying, "You know we have a counseling center here on campus, where you can get help for free. Talking about your anxiety and finding ways to manage it will likely help you feel better and more in control of your emotions." Gauge the student's reaction and offer to help make the phone call for an initial appointment.

The higher education professional can prepare the student for the types of interventions that may be suggested by a mental health professional. Counseling can include strategies to combat negative beliefs and may also involve biofeedback. Biofeedback can be conducted in most campus counseling centers and includes specialized equipment that measures such signals as brain activity, blood pressure, muscle tension, heart rate, and skin temperature. Through biofeedback, the student learns to become aware of their physiological responses and ultimately control them. In an ethnically diverse population of college students, biofeedback combined with traditional counseling has been found to significantly reduce students' anxiety and stress beyond counseling alone (Ratanasiripong et al., 2012). Mental health professionals will work with students to challenge maladaptive cognitions through a form of treatment called cognitive-behavioral therapy, or CBT. These techniques assist students in evaluating their thoughts and beliefs and forming more realistic appraisals. The mental health professional will help the student challenge and change unhelpful cognitive distortions and behaviors, improve their ability to regulate their emotions, and develop personal coping strategies.

An evaluation by a mental health professional can determine the best course of treatment. CBT is most often used for anxiety disorders; however, some students may require medication to reduce their anxiety in order to benefit from counseling. A student with panic attacks may require medication to alleviate the intense anxiety that accompanies these episodes. For many people who struggle with panic, just knowing that they may rely on medication for their symptoms is a relief. For those students with social anxiety or phobias, more intensive, extended treatment with a professional may be required. The social demands of college may be overwhelming for the student with social anxiety, causing them to consider dropping out. Interventions can provide strategies to help these students manage their feelings and beliefs.

When students present with test anxiety, it is important to get a determination of whether they may have a learning disability that is contributing to these feelings. In cases of a suspected learning disability, a referral to the disability resource office may be warranted. Inquiring about whether a student had an individualized learning plan during school, prior to college, can be a good starting place. While colleges are not mandated to offer the same services, they do have resources and advisors available. A student who constantly struggles with assignments, has difficulty understanding directions, and seems unable to keep up in lectures may have an underlying learning disability. These students may be able to receive accommodations such as extended time on tests, which may assist in alleviating anxiety about having enough time to finish (Nelson et al., 2015). Other services include a note taker, use of a laptop in class or access to recorded lectures, or flexible deadlines for work.

Conclusion

Anxiety is a common experience for many students, and moderate levels can be motivating. Concern about an upcoming test will motivate students to set aside time to study and prepare. However, when anxiety becomes intense and interferes with daily functioning, students can become overwhelmed and experience disruptive physical symptoms. For some students, engaging in mindfulness and physical exercise may be enough to handle these feelings, but other students may require the help of a counselor or medication. Stress is a universal experience for college students who may worry about their grades, making friends, and being away from home. How students handle stress is important, and the higher education professional may be able to offer guidance on healthy coping strategies. Learning about healthy relationships, developing time management skills, and working toward a work–life balance at school are good starting points.

References

Aaron, R. E., Rinehart, K. L., & Ceballos, N. A. (2011). Arts-based interventions to reduce anxiety levels among college students, *Arts & Health*, *3*(1), 27–38. https://doi.org/10.1080/17533015.2010.481290

American College Health Association. (2022). *American College Health Association–National College Health Assessment III: Reference group executive summary fall 2021.* https://www.acha.org/documents/ncha/NCHA-III_ FALL_2021_REFERENCE_GROUP_EXECUTIVE_SUMMARY.pdf

Bamber, M. D., & Kraenzle Schneider, J. (2016). Mindfulness-based meditation to decrease stress and anxiety in college students: A narrative synthesis of the research. *Educational Research Review*, *18*, 1–32. https://doi.org/10.1016/j.edurev.2015.12.004

Bamber, M. D., & Morpeth, E. (2019). Effects of mindfulness meditation on college student anxiety: A meta-analysis. *Mindfulness*, *10*(2), 203–214. https://doi.org/10.1007/S12671-018-0965-5

Chappell, M. S., Blanding, Z. B., Silverstein, M. E., Takahashi, M., Newman, B., Gubi, A., & McCann, N. (2005). Test anxiety and academic performance in undergraduate and graduate students. *Journal of Educational Psychology*, *97*(2), 268–274. https://doi.org/10.1037/0022-0663.97.2.268

Cheung, K., Tam, K. Y., Tsang, M. H., Zhang, L. W., & Lit, S. W. (2020). Depression, anxiety and stress in different subgroups of first-year university students from 4-year cohort data. *Journal of Affective Disorders*, *274*, 305–314. https://doi.org/10.1016/j.jad.2020.05.041

College Parents of America. (2019, January 3). *5 main causes of stress for college students.* https://collegeparents.org/2019/01/03/5-main-causes-of-stress-for-college-students%ef%bb%bf

Conley, K. M., & Lehman, B. J. (2012). Test anxiety and cardiovascular responses to daily academic stressors. *Stress and Health: Journal of the International Society for the Investigation of Stress*, *28*(1), 41–50. https://doi.org/10.1002/smi.1399

Eustis, E. H., Hayes-Skelton, S. A., Orsillo, S. M., & Roemer, L. (2018). Surviving and thriving during stress: A randomized clinical trial comparing a brief web-based therapist-assisted acceptance-based behavioral intervention versus waitlist control for college students. *Behavior Therapy*, *49*(6), 889–903. https://doi.org/10.1016/j.beth.2018.05.009

Galloway Burke, M., Sauerheber, J., Hughey, A., & Laves, K. (2017). *Helping skills for working with college students.* Routledge.

Gerwing, T. G., Rash, J. A., Gerwing, A. M. A., Bramble, B., & Landine, J. (2015). Perceptions and incidence of test anxiety. *The Canadian Journal for Scholarship of Teaching and Learning*, *6*(3), Article 3. https://doi.org/10.5206/cjsotl-rcacea.2015.3.3

Hirokawa, K., Yagi, A., & Miyata, Y. (2002). An examination of the effects of stress management training for Japanese college students of social work. *International Journal of Stress Management, 9*(2), 113–123.

Hughes, B. M. (2004). Academic study, college examinations, and stress: Issues in the interpretation of cardiovascular reactivity assessments with student participants. *Journal of Applied Biobehavioral Research, 9*(1), 23–44. https://doi.org/10.1111/j.1751-9861.2004.tb00090.x

Hughes, B. M. (2005). Study, examinations, and stress: Blood pressure assessments in college students. *Educational Review, 57*(1), 21–36. https://doi.org/10.1080/0013191042000274169

Mahmoud, J. S. R., Staten, R. T., Hall, L. A., & Lennie, T. A. (2012). The relationship among young adult college students' depression, anxiety, stress, demographics, life satisfaction, and coping styles. *Issues in Mental Health Nursing, 33*(3), 149–156. https://doi.org/10.3109/01612840.2011.632708

Moore, K., & Craciun G. (2020). Fear of missing out and personality predictors of social networking sites usage: The Instagram case. *Psychological Reports, 124*(4), 1761–1787. https://doi.org/10.1177/0033294120936184

National Center for Education Statistics. (2019). *Table 503.40: Percentage of 16- to 64-year-old undergraduate students who were employed, by attendance status, hours worked per week, and selected characteristics: 2000, 2010, and 2018* (Digest of Education Statistics, 2019). https://nces.ed.gov/programs/digest/d19/tables/dt19_503.40.asp

Nelson, J. M., Lindstrom, W., & Foels, P. A. (2015). Test anxiety among college students with specific reading disability (dyslexia): Nonverbal ability and working memory as predictors. *Journal of Learning Disabilities, 48*(4), 422–432. https://doi.org/10.1177/0022219413507604

Pelletier, J. E., Lytle, L. A., & Laska, M. N. (2016). Stress, health risk behaviors, and weight status among community college students. *Health Education & Behavior, 43*(2), 139–144. https://doi.org/10.1177%2F1090198115598983

Price, M., Hides, L., Cockshaw, W., Staneva, A. A., & Stoyanov, S. R. (2016). Young love: Romantic concerns and associated mental health issues among adolescent help-seekers. *Behavioral Sciences, 6*(2), 1–14. https://doi.org/10.3390/bs6020009

Putwain, D. W., Connors, L., & Symes, W. (2010). Do cognitive distortions mediate the test anxiety–examination performance relationship? *Educational Psychology, 30*, 11–26. https://doi.org/10.1080/01443410903328866

Ratanasiripong, P., Sverduk, K., Prince, J., & Hayashino, D. (2012). Biofeedback and counseling for stress and anxiety among students. *Journal of College Student Development, 53*(5), 742–749. https://doi.org/10.1353/csd.2012.0070

Shankar N., & Park, C. (2016). Effects of stress on students' physical and mental health and academic success. *International Journal of School & Educational Psychology, 4*(1), 5–9. https://doi.org/10.1080/21683603.2016.1130532

Spielberger, C. D., Anton, W. D., & Bedell, J. (2015). The nature and treatment of test anxiety. In M. Zuckerman & C. D. Spielberger (Eds.), *Emotions and anxiety: New concepts, methods, and applications* (pp. 317–344). Psychology Press. https://doi.org/10.4324/9781315744643

Sprung, J. M., & Rogers, A. (2020). Work-life balance as a predictor of college student anxiety and depression. *Journal of American College Health, 69*(7), 775–782. https://doi.org/10.1080/07448481.2019.1706540

Sun, J., & Hagedorn, L. S. (2016). Homesickness at college: Its impact on academic performance and retention. *Journal of College Student Development, 57*(8), 943–957. https://doi.org/10.1353/csd.2016.0092

Tripathi, K., & Sharma, K. (2013). Causes of academic stress among college students and its managements. *Indian Journal of Health and Wellbeing, 4*(5), 1161–1164.

Watson J., & Faucher, A. (2020). Stress and anxiety. In D. Paladino, L. Gonzalez, & J. Watson (Eds.), *College counseling and student development: Theory, practice and campus collaboration* (pp. 331–352). American Counseling Association.

CHAPTER 8

Depression and Suicide

According to the American College Health Association (2022) National College Health Assessment, the rates of students struggling with depression and suicidal thoughts continue to rise. In 2022, 29% of respondents had considered suicide and 3% had made an attempt; 12% had engaged in self-injury; 27% reported feeling depressed; and another 80% reported feeling moderately or severely stressed within the previous 30 days. These rates show not only an increase from the 2019 survey, but an even more dramatic one from the 2012 survey. This chapter discusses the signs and symptoms of depression and suicidal thinking, and how to recognize them in students. Given the potential lethality of severe depression, it is critical that higher education professionals be ready to assist the student and make appropriate interventions. The chapter also includes skills to approach and discuss these sensitive issues with students who might be struggling.

Basic Signs and Symptoms of Depression and Suicide

Students struggling with depression and suicidal thoughts continue to be a major concern on college campuses, and suicide is one of the leading causes of death among college-aged students (Centers for Disease Control and Prevention [CDC], 2022a). In 2021, according to a nationwide study by The Healthy Minds Network, an estimated 13% of college students reported experiencing suicidal ideation in the previous year. This number is higher than previous estimates of suicidal ideation ranging from 6% to 12% (Arria et al., 2009; Brener et al., 1999; Garlow et al., 2008; Kisch et al., 2005; Wilcox et al., 2010). Suicide is the second leading of cause of death among traditional-aged college students (CDC, 2020). Despite efforts on campuses across the country, these numbers are not improving. With the dramatic increase from 2012 to 2022 in rates of students struggling with suicidal thoughts and depression, higher education professionals need to continue to find ways to reach out to students, offer help, and lower these numbers. One way to do this is by understanding the signs, symptoms, and most effective methods to approach and talk to students who might be struggling.

Depression

One of the main challenges of dealing with depression is being able to distinguish between sadness and clinical depression. Understanding this difference is critical so higher education professionals can know when to be concerned. Members of the university community often struggle with this distinction, which means they can miss key signs of a student struggling with something more significant. Many of the issues discussed in this book can cause confusion for noncounselors, because the behaviors that signal a need for attention can also straddle the norm. Table 8.1 delineates

> **Case Study**
>
> Chris is a freshman who lives in a residence hall on campus. At the beginning of the year, he was fairly involved with student clubs and active in his classes. He seemed to be adjusting well to college life. Lately, he has seemed more withdrawn. He hasn't shown up to programs, he doesn't come out of his room much, and his hallmates say they rarely see him in class. At first, they thought maybe he was just upset because his girlfriend had broken up with him and he was struggling in his classes, but as weeks passed their concern has deepened. They are worried about him but don't want to bother him. They have tried to encourage him to come with them to parties or the dining hall, but he says no. They finally told the resident assistant (RA). The RA talked with Chris, who mentioned the breakup and his classes but then really didn't seem to want to talk anymore. He said things like, "It doesn't really matter; I'm not sure I'll be here next semester anyhow." He ended the conversation with, "It's OK. I'm fine."

what to look for to help distinguish normal sadness from more concerning signs of depression.

The commonly used book to help diagnose mental conditions, the American Psychiatric Association's (2013) *Diagnostic and Statistical Manual of Mental Disorders, Fifth Edition* (*DSM-5*), defines *depression* as a common and serious mood disorder. Affected students experience symptoms such as hopelessness and sadness, and they lose interest in activities they used to enjoy. Often, as we see with our case study, students who are struggling with depression demonstrate a marked departure in their behavior. Chris's friends and hallmates noticed that he had stopped joining them in activities and in the dining hall, and he seemed to be withdrawing. If this

Table 8.1
Sadness versus Depression

Sadness	Depression
A typical human emotion	A medical mental illness
Typically happens in response to an event	Often no cause or trigger
Allows daily functioning to continue	Causes difficulty in school, relationships, and daily life
Is usually short-lived and fades with time	Often takes professional intervention/treatment, such as therapy or medication, to improve

behavior had been consistent since the semester began, it would be less concerning. As the *DSM-5* mentions, a major sign of depression is diminished interest and pleasure in most activities, as well as a depressed mood for most of the day. Students suffering from depression will often stop their usual activities. Their sleep is often impacted—they are getting either too much or too little. They may seem tired or have less energy. They might have a diminished ability to think or concentrate, which can have a negative impact on classes, as we see with Chris. They may also experience feelings of worthlessness or guilt. Other signs include irritability, negative moods or brooding, and obsessive rumination and worry. Depression can often be accompanied by feelings of anxiety as well as complaints about declining physical health or pain. Many students experience some of these feelings at one point or another in their lives; these are not uncommon emotions. The main difference, however, is that for a student experiencing depression, these symptoms last for an extended period of time. To be considered diagnosable depression, these symptoms need to persist for at least 2 weeks.

Higher education professionals will often ask how to distinguish depression from sadness. Because many of the symptoms of depression mimic sadness, it can be challenging to determine the student's condition. A good rule of thumb is assessing the combination of factors and the extent to which they are affecting the student's ability to function and handle daily activities and tasks. Another factor is recognizing that sadness often has a trigger: a specific event, person, or situation that can bring about these feelings. Typically, depression occurs with no known reason; students suffering from depression will often have these feelings about most things in their lives (Psycom, 2022). Often, the people around the depressed student think that everything about their life looks perfect and that they *should* be happy. If the student's symptoms persist, the higher education professional should be concerned and prepared to intervene.

Another effective tool to use when assessing a student is the mnemonic IS PATH WARM (see Figure 8.1). This can be used to determine if a student is at risk for suicide. These warning signs were compiled by a task force of expert clinical-researchers and put into this format for the general public to use, to make it easier to distinguish signs and symptoms that may precede suicide (Juhnke et al., 2007).

Figure 8.1
IS PATH WARM

Ideation
Substance Abuse

Purposelessness
Anxiety
Trapped
Hopelessness

Withdrawal
Anger
Recklessness
Mood Change

Bipolar Disorder

Bipolar disorder is one of the most common types of mood disorders. It is characterized by "manic/depressive" episodes, where the student will go from periods of extreme highs to extreme lows. A student in a manic phase will often appear overly hyper, even as if on a "high." They may seem overconfident or have an unrealistic sense of self-entitlement or inflated self-esteem. The student will be on the go, often staying up late and forgoing sleep, feeling rested after as little as 3 hours each night. When asked about this behavior, they might claim they are so busy getting schoolwork done or pursuing another goal they just cannot stop. Often a student in a manic phase will engage in risky behavior such as spending sprees, increased substance abuse, and unsafe sex practices. These periods can last up to a week and are then followed by a depressive state, which can last up to 2 weeks.

Bipolar disorder is an important condition for higher education administrators to learn about and understand, as this condition often first emerges in students during college (Simon & Lejeune, 2011). In a 10,000-student university, one can expect one or two cases of the first episode of mania per year (Kennedy et al., 2005). The student's behavior will appear "off," or not quite right, to their friends. It will be important to get the student to the campus counseling center as soon as possible.

Suicide

As seen from the American College Health Association (2022) data, the numbers regarding depression and suicide are concerning—the trend is continuing upward, despite numerous efforts on college campuses aimed at prevention and stigma reduction. Suicide rates among students are alarming, demonstrating that there is still much to be understood about the signs and symptoms, how best to intervene, and who seems to be the most affected. Research has demonstrated that race, gender, and sexual orientation are associated with suicide risk in the general population. Men tend to die by suicide more often than women do, but women make more attempts (Beautrais, 2003; Nock et al., 2008). Non-Hispanic Whites and nonheterosexuals are at higher risk than their White, heterosexual peers (Figueiredo & Abreu, 2015; Nock et al., 2008), but less is known about how these cultural factors predict suicidal behavior in college students (Coduti et al., 2016). Students with disabilities tend to have more suicidal thoughts than those without (Coduti et al., 2016).

Suicide is one of the most difficult topics to discuss for many people, both on and off campus, and it can be intimidating to raise it with students. It is important to understand that suicidal thoughts and behaviors exist on a continuum, ranging from passive to active, and moving from passing thoughts to plans, gestures, attempts, and completions. It is not uncommon for students to have passing thoughts of ending their lives without ever having any intention to act on those thoughts. Suicidal thinking becomes more concerning when it is persistent and driven by increased emotional distress. The student's thoughts might be directed toward how and when they might kill themselves, and actual gestures or attempts elevate the overall level of risk.

Triggering life events can increase a student's risk for suicide, and often there are aspects of the college experience that become risk factors as well. These events usually involve some sort of loss for the student. Additional events can also include role changes, academic demands, career indecision, financial pressures, and loneliness and separation from support networks (Hirsch & Ellis, 1996; Martin et al., 2005).

In Chris's case, the breakup with his girlfriend may have been the precipitating event. Other events could include the death of a loved one; the loss of a position on campus, such as a leadership role in a club or organization or a position on an athletic team; a traumatic experience; a major breakup; or being placed on academic probation or getting academically dismissed. Being aware of these events can help higher education professionals intervene before something tragic might occur.

> **Case Study**
>
> Juan has been playing soccer for as long as he can remember. As he got older, he worked even harder to earn a college scholarship. He achieved that goal and began college (at his first-choice school) on a full soccer scholarship. His first year went smoothly. Juan bonded well with his teammates, did well academically, and felt well connected to the institution. In the fall of his sophomore year, he suffered a severe injury that ended his ability to play soccer. His full athletic scholarship was in jeopardy and would most likely be taken away. Juan fell into a deep depression, he began isolating from his teammates and friends, and his grades dropped. He has been heard making comments like, "Well, I won't be here next semester anyhow."

Juan's case illustrates the complexities of identifying what might trigger a depressive or suidical episode. Juan's entire identity has been shaken, and he is facing the possibility of having to leave the school where he had been so successful. His behavior and comment are concerning and worth follow-up. His comment is unclear and needs to be explored. His situation is the type that could put a student into a suicidal state, and it would be important for higher education administrators to check in and follow up as well as offer guidance.

Being in college is actually a protective factor against suicide, with social support often cited as key to reducing suicide and suicide ideation (Kleiman et al., 2014; Klonsky & May, 2015). The CDC (2022b) has promoted "healthy connectedness" as a strategic direction for suicide prevention. Data show that students in college are less likely to commit suicide than their noncollege peers (Drum et al., 2009). Human beings have a strong "fight or flight" instinct, and it is not easy for them to take their own lives. The act of suicide often comes with great ambivalence. The harder it is to complete the act, the less likely it is to happen. College campuses, on the most basic level, provide restricted access to the lethal means needed to complete a suicide. Students also have access to effective clinical interventions and support for help-seeking. Interventions in counseling centers are often free and are always confidential. College campuses provide students with a community of support and connection. Students are surrounded by faculty, staff, and other students who provide connection, care, and ongoing support. This concept of social support is particularly relevant in the college setting because students are often in situations where they are living and working with their peers in a community environment, which increases their sense of belonging and connectedness (Lamis et al., 2016). Furthermore, campus professionals have been increasing their focus on improving skills in problem solving, conflict resolution, and nonviolent ways of handling disputes. This does not mean, however, that students do not continue to struggle with issues of depression and suicide.

Students turn to their friends, a family member, or a trusted faculty or staff member when they are in crisis, such as feeling suicidal. According to a 2009 survey of undergraduate students by mtvU and the Associated Press, when asked who they turn to when they are upset, 76% answered they would turn to friends for help and 63% said their parents. They were far less likely to seek professional help, with only 20% saying they would turn to campus counseling. This held true in The Healthy Minds Network 2021 study, where 41% said they would turn to a friend, 37% said a family member, and 30% said a significant other. But only 4% chose a faculty member, and only 2% said they would opt for a staff member. But students are still struggling in high numbers—in that same mtvU and Associated Press (2009) poll, 9% indicated "serious" thoughts of harming themselves in the past year, and half of those considered talking to a professional. Of those who talked to non-professionals, only 52% found it helpful. Those numbers are alarming and show that higher education professionals are unprepared to help when approached with issues as serious as depression and potential suicide.

Approaching the Student

Approaching a student who is depressed and potentially suicidal can be intimidating. Higher education professionals often share that one of their biggest fears is simply saying the wrong thing, and that fear often leads them to do or say nothing. While this response is understandable, it can lead to the student feeling even further isolated and alone. Providing someone with the opportunity to talk about their suicidal thinking is, in most cases, a great relief. Use of empathy and nonjudgmental responding is very helpful. With the students in both case studies, it would be helpful to ask direct questions, such as "Tell me what you mean when you say 'you're not sure you'll be here next semester'" or "Are you thinking about hurting yourself?" Another good approach is saying something like, "Sometimes when things are not going well and someone feels down, they think about hurting themselves. Are you having any thoughts like that?" This can normalize the feelings for the person. When engaging with students, it is important to focus on the behaviors that are alarming. It is also essential to instill hope. Students who are depressive or suicidal often lack hope and cannot see that their situation will change or improve. It is often said that suicide is a permanent solution to a temporary problem. But, unfortunately, the person struggling cannot see that. Saying something like, "I know you do not have hope right now, but I will hold the hope for you until you are ready" can be just what the student needs to get them through the crisis. This statement gives students the sense that while they may not have hope, the higher education professional has the confidence their situation will improve. This is a common suicide

Depression and Suicide 97

prevention tool that can help a student condidering suicide see that there is hope, even if they are not feeling it themselves.

The following are some guidelines to consider when approaching a student you might be concerned about:

1. **Plan a time and place.** This is an important conversation. You want to make sure you have enough time to give the conversation the attention it deserves, so plan accordingly. Pick a place where you have privacy and the student will feel comfortable to talk freely.
2. **Choose your approach—direct or indirect.** As discussed, asking a student if they are contemplating suicide **will not** increase their risk for suicide. Giving them the opportunity to discuss their feelings will often provide relief, not increase their distress.
   - Less direct approaches:
     - Have you been unhappy lately?
     - You know, when people are as upset as you seem to be, they sometimes wish they were dead; I'm wondering if you're feeling that way too?
     - You seem pretty miserable; can you tell me more about how you're feeling?
   - Direct approaches:
     - Have you thought about hurting yourself?
     - Have you ever wanted to stop living?
     - Are you thinking about suicide?
3. **Listen and ask to help.**
   - Listen to the student with an open mind, using empathy and nonjudgment.
   - Wait until the student is done speaking before responding.
   - Be OK with some silence.

- Ask the student if they will go with you to see a counselor or if they will let you help them make an appointment to see a counselor.

In all of these scenarios, you want the student to know that you are there for them, and that they are not alone. While you do not want to try to fix their problems, letting them know there are solutions other than suicide can be helpful. Assuring them that they will not always feel this way is a good first step. Getting them to counseling is another critical step in the process. Once you complete this "warm handoff" to counseling, reassure the student that you will still be there to support them.

Campus Response

There is evidence that mental health counseling can alleviate the impact of depression and suicidal thinking (Schwartz, 2013). While these benefits may be somewhat attributed to the self-seeking nature of those who go for help, it is still essential that campuses continue to raise awareness about this important resource. Despite efforts, a very small number of college students—just 26%—are aware of the mental health services available to them (Westefeld et al., 2005).

As a result, many campuses have tried to implement programming aimed at increasing help-seeking behaviors and getting students to seek treatment in campus counseling centers (Garlow et al., 2008; Haas et al., 2008). While programs have traditionally focused on training faculty and staff, research has shown that students overwhelming turn to peers. Drum et al. (2009) found that among students with serious suicidal ideation and attempts, 46% said they never talked to anyone else about these issues, and of those students who did talk to someone else, 67% of the time it was a peer, most often a close friend or roommate. Furthermore, students with suicidal ideation were more reticent to seek professional help than those who were struggling with mental health concerns without suicidal ideation.

Professionals within college counseling and health and wellness centers can take initiative and assume leadership in the strategic design and implementation of interventions to improve overall student support, safety, and well-being. However, many counseling center staff see themselves in more traditional clinical roles, providing professional mental health assessment and treatment and occasional training and outreach programming. Under the weight of ever-increasing student requests for services (Gallagher, 2012), a call for more clinical staff is often counseling centers' first reaction. But with the prevalence of mental health distress on college campuses, no counseling center could ever meet the clinical needs of all students. New paradigms of treatment and community intervention need to be investigated and developed to address the overall mental health needs of the campus community. Fortunately, much has been learned over the past decade, and college campuses have adopted public health models for suicide prevention and mental health promotion. This work has been largely supported by the Garrett Lee Smith Memorial Act of Congress in 2004, which under the guidance of the federal Substance Abuse and Mental Health Services Administration (SAMHSA) has authorized colleges to study and develop best practices in campus suicide prevention and mental health promotion. Each year, SAMHSA awards substantial grants to 30 or more institutions across the United States. The Act also funded the creation of the Suicide Prevention Resource Center, a clearinghouse for information and research and a major provider of technical support for college campuses invested in initiatives to promote mental health and prevent suicide.

In providing leadership for mental health education and promotion activities, counseling centers must involve the entire campus community. Such efforts will build trusting connections among helping resources and encourage conversations about mental health issues that can reduce mental health stigma.

Conclusion

Despite increased efforts by colleges and universities, the numbers of students struggling with depression and suicidal thoughts continue to rise. The more comfortable and confident higher education professionals feel in addressing and responding to students in distress, the more they will be able to encourage students to get the help they need. One of the most important things a higher education professional can do is to show empathy and understanding, and let students know they are not alone in their feelings. Providing a listening ear and a sense of hope can go a long way in helping students take the first step toward getting the support they need. Higher education professional are often insecure about their abilities to have these sensitive and difficult conversations, often fearing they will only make the situation worse. Once they feel empowered, armed with solid training and concrete steps to take, they can move forward knowing their interventions can make a big difference in the outcomes for students.

References

American College Health Association. (2012). *American College Health Association–National College Health Assessment II: Reference group executive summary spring 2012.* https://www.acha.org/documents/ncha/ACHA-NCHA-II_ReferenceGroup_ExecutiveSummary_Spring2012.pdf

American College Health Association. (2019). *American College Health Association–National College Health Assessment III: Reference group executive summary fall 2019.* https://www.acha.org/documents/ncha/NCHA-III_Fall_2019_Reference_Group_Executive_Summary_updated.pdf

American College Health Association. (2022). *American College Health Association–National College Health Assessment III: Reference group executive summary spring 2022.* https://www.acha.org/documents/ncha/NCHA-III_SPRING_2022_REFERENCE_GROUP_EXECUTIVE_SUMMARY.pdf

American Psychiatric Association. (2013). *Diagnostic and statistical manual of mental disorders* (5th ed.). https://doi.org/10.1176/appi.books.9780890425596

Arria, A. M., O'Grady, K. E., Caldeira, K. M., Vincent, K. B., Wilcox, H. C., & Wish, E. D. (2009). Suicide ideation among college students: A multivariate analysis. *Archives of Suicide Research, 13,* 230–246. https://doi.org/10.1080/13811110903044351

Beautrais, A. (2003). Suicide and serious suicide attempts in youth: A multiple-group comparison study. *The American Journal of Psychiatry, 160,* 1093–1099. https://doi.org/10.1176/appi.ajp.160.6.1093

Brener, N. D., Hassan, S. S., & Barrios, L. C. (1999). Suicidal ideation among college students in the United States. *Journal of Consulting and Clinical Psychology, 67*(6), 1004–1008. https://doi.org/10.1037/0022-006X.67.6.1004

Centers for Disease Control and Prevention. (2022a, October 24). *Facts about suicide.* https://www.cdc.gov/suicide/facts/index.html

Centers for Disease Control and Prevention. (2022b, August 25). *School connectedness.* https://www.cdc.gov/healthyschools/school_connectedness.htm

Coduti, W. A., Hayes, J. A., Locke, B. D., & Youn, S. J. (2016). Mental health and professional help-seeking among college students with disabilities. *Rehabilitation Psychology, 61*(3), 288–296. https://doi.org/10.1037/rep0000101

Drum, D. J., Brownson, C., Denmark, A. B., & Smith, S. E. (2009). New data on the nature of suicidal crises in college students: Shifting the paradigm. *Professional Psychology: Research and Practice, 40*(3), 213–222. https://doi.org/10.1037/a0014465

Figueiredo, A., & Abreu, T. (2015). Suicide among LGBT individuals. *European Psychiatry, 30*(S1), 1815. https://doi.org/10.1016/S0924-9338(15)31398-5

Gallagher, R. P. (2012). *National survey of counseling center directors 2011: Project report.* International Association of Counseling Services.

Garlow, S. J., Rosenberg, J., Moore, J., Haas, A. P., Koestner, B., Hendin, H., & Nemeroff, C. (2008). Depression, desperation, and suicidal ideation in college students: Results from the American Foundation for Suicide Prevention College Screening Project at Emory University. *Depression and Anxiety, 25,* 482–488. https://doi.org/10.1002/da.20321

Haas, A., Koestner, B., Rosenberg, J., Moore, D., Garlow, S. J., Sedway, J., & Nemeroff, C. B. (2008). An interactive web-based method of outreach to college students at risk for suicide. *Journal of American College Health, 57,* 15–22. https://doi.org/10.3200/jach.57.1.15-22

The Healthy Minds Network. (2021). *The healthy minds study 2021 winter/spring data report.* https://healthymindsnetwork.org/wp-content/uploads/2022/01/HMS_nationalwinter2021_-update1.5.21.pdf

Hirsch, J. K., & Ellis, J. B. (1996). Differences in life stress and reasons for living among college suicide ideators and non-ideators. *College Student Journal, 30*(3), 377–386.

Juhnke, G. A., Granello, P. F., & Lebrón-Striker, M. A. (2007). *IS PATH WARM? A suicide assessment mnemonic for counselors (ACAPCD-03).* American Counseling Association.

Kennedy, N., Everitt, B., Boydell, J., Van Os, J., Jones, P. B., & Murray, R. M. (2005). Incidence and distribution of first-episode mania by age: Results from a 35-year study. *Psychological Medicine, 35*(6), 855–863. https://doi.org/10.1017/s0033291704003307

Kisch, J., Leino, E. V., & Silverman, M. M. (2005). Aspects of suicidal behavior, depression, and treatment in college students: Results from the spring 2000 National College Health Assessment Survey. *Suicide & Life-Threatening Behavior, 35*(1), 3–13. https://doi.org/10.1521/suli.35.1.3.59263

Kleiman, E. M., Riskind, J. H., & Schaefer, K. E. (2014). Social support and positive events as suicide resiliency factors: Examination of synergistic buffering effects. *Archives of Suicide Research, 18*, 144–155. https://doi.org/10.1080/13811118.2013.826155

Klonsky, E. D., & May, A. M. (2015). The three-step theory (3ST): A new theory of suicide rooted in the "ideation-to-action" framework. *International Journal of Cognitive Therapy, 8*, 114–129. https://doi.org/10.1521/ijct.2015.8.2.114

Lamis, A., Ballard., E. D., May, A. M., & Dvorak, R. D. (2016). Depressive symptoms and suicidal ideation in college students: The mediating and moderating roles of hopelessness, alcohol problems, and social support. *Journal of Clinical Psychology, 72*(9), 919–932. https://doi.org/10.1002/jclp.22295

Martin, G., Richardson, A. S., Bergen, H. A., Roeger, L., & Allison, S. (2005). Perceived academic performance, self-esteem and locus of control as indicators of need for assessment of adolescent suicide risk: Implications for teachers. *Journal of Adolescence, 28*(1), 75–87. https://doi.org/10.1016/j.adolescence.2004.04.005

mtvU & Associated Press. (2009, May 21). *New mtvU & Associated Press poll shows how stress, the economy & other factors are affecting college students' mental health* [Press release]. https://www.bloomberg.com/press-releases/2009-05-21/new-mtvu-associated-press-poll-shows-how-stress-the-economy

Nock, M. K., Borges, G., Bromet, E. J., Cha, C. B., Kessler, R. C., & Lee, S. (2008). Suicide and suicidal behavior. *Epidemiologic Reviews, 30*(1), 133–154. https://doi.org/10.1093/epirev/mxn002

Psycom. (2022, June 8). *Depression definition and DSM-5 diagnostic criteria.* https://www.psycom.net/depression-definition-dsm-5-diagnostic-criteria

Schwartz, A. J. (2013). Comparing the risk of suicide of college students with nonstudents. *Journal of College Student Psychotherapy, 27*(2), 120–137. https://doi.org/10.1080/87568225.2013.766108

Simon, M. W., & Lejeune, M. D. (2011). Special considerations in the treatment of college students with bipolar disorder. *Journal of American College Health, 59*(7), 666–669. https://doi.org/10.1080/07448481.2010.528100

Westefeld, J. S., Homaifar, B., Spotts, J., Furr, S., Range, L., & Worth, J. L. (2005). Perceptions concerning college student suicide: Data from four universities. *Suicide and Life Threatening Behavior, 35*(6), 640–645. https://doi.org/10.1521/suli.2005.35.6.640

Wilcox, H. C., Arria, A. M., Caldeira, K. M., Vincent, K. B., Pinchevsky, G. M., & O'Grady, K. E. (2010). Prevalence and predictors of persistent suicide ideation, plans, and attempts during college. *Journal of Affective Disorders, 127*(1–3), 287–294. https://doi.org/10.1016/j.jad.2010.04.017

CHAPTER 9

Eating Disorders

This chapter presents a current, literature-informed discussion of eating disorders in young adults. Readers will learn the signs and symptoms of commonly seen eating disorders and how to recognize them. Given the secrecy and denial that often accompany these conditions, this chapter will guide readers on how to approach students about whom they have a concern. Because some eating disorders can be fatal, an emphasis will be placed on the seriousness of these conditions.

Basic Signs and Symptoms of Eating Disorders

Society places great emphasis on appearance and weight. Diets seem to dominate the media, with messages about eating healthy and avoiding certain foods. As medicine advances, people are more concerned about living longer and staying in shape. Such interest in fitness and health is obviously beneficial; however, many young people have developed an unhealthy attention to their bodies and food intake.

The transition to college can be considered a risk period for the development of disordered eating. Because body image dissatisfaction, preoccupation with weight, and unhealthy weight management (all hallmarks of eating disorders) are common among normal-weight college students (Schwitzer et al., 1998), detecting an eating disorder can often be difficult. Different kinds of disordered eating typically occur during the young adult years, with the average age of onset for most eating disorders being 14 to 22 years (Rohde et al., 2017). The astute professional needs training in order to distinguish "normal" eating patterns from those that are "abnormal."

Case Study

> Sasha seems to have made a good transition to her first year of college. She has friends, is doing well in her classes, and has found a part-time job at the campus coffee shop. Her parents are a bit surprised when they see her at home for fall break. Sasha wears baggy sweatpants and sweatshirts most of the time, but she appears to have lost a lot of weight. Sasha denies the weight loss and tells her parents that she is just a bit stressed about classes. Her friends have also noticed that she tends to eat little at meals and pushes the food around her plate. When they ask her about her eating habits, she always has the same reply: "I'm not that hungry. I just ate at the coffee shop." In fact, Sasha is rarely eating. She often skips meals and works out excessively. She has lost about 20 pounds, and because she is only 5 feet, 5 inches tall, this amount of weight loss looks drastic.

Such behavior as late-night snacking while studying, after-dinner pizza orders, and ordering food delivery after midnight is considered typical among college students; however, disordered eating among this cohort does occur. The range of disordered eating behavior can include fad diets (e.g., Atkins, paleo, grapefruit), "clean" eating (e.g., restricting fats, dairy, or gluten), over-exercising, abusing laxatives, and occasional bingeing and/or purging. All are concerning behaviors, but they do not meet the criteria for an eating disorder. Sometimes initial attempts to eat healthy may lead to choosing restrictive diets, skipping meals, and taking diet pills and may potentially progress to diagnosable eating disorders (Golden et al., 2016; Lebow et al., 2015). Some of these symptoms are seen in Sasha, including skipping meals and overexercising, which has led to concerning weight loss. It is important that higher education professionals evaluate the impact that eating behaviors have on the student's life: Are they restricting where the student can go, forcing them to withdraw from social activities and count calories all day long? If so, these may be signs of a more serious condition.

Although disordered eating can occur at any age, college students tend to be particularly vulnerable to it (Zotter & Reel, 2013). Franko et al. (2005) estimated that between 10% and 30% of college women appear to be at risk for developing an eating disorder over the course of their college years. A survey administered by the American College Health Association (ACHA, 2022) found that 5% of college students reported being diagnosed with an eating disorder at some time in their life. Social pressure to be thin and a desire to "fit in" and have body shapes extolled in the media likely promote body dissatisfaction and compel weight-loss efforts (Derenne & Beresin, 2018). Women under 20 appear to be affected by eating disorders at dramatically higher rates than those of the general population (Hudson et al., 2007). Using the most recent criteria for eating disorders in the *Diagnostic and Statistical Manual of Mental Disorders, Fifth Edition* (*DSM-5*), Stice et al. (2013) found a lifetime prevalence of eating disorders of 13% among this population, concluding that "one in eight young women" (p. 455) will have some form of a diagnosable eating disorder.

College students may be at particular risk for disordered eating and body dissatisfaction due to weight gain that frequently takes place during this stage of life (Hoffman et al., 2006). Often referred to as the "freshman 15" is the prevailing belief that when students go away to college for the first time, they will gain weight. In fact, some students gain weight (on average 10 pounds), but some students lose weight, and others maintain their weight (Carithers-Thomas et al., 2010). Many factors contribute to this weight gain, including new eating patterns, increased alcohol intake, decreased physical activity, stress or emotional eating, and snacking more regularly. This weight gain, or fear of gaining weight, can be a trigger for some students to begin dieting and take other measures to control their weight, and these choices may turn unhealthy.

Case Study

Jamie was delighted when she was offered a spot in the sorority of her choice. She was happy to have gained a group of girlfriends and an active social calendar. As soon as a room opened in the sorority house, she moved in. Jamie enjoyed having a bunch of "sisters" with whom she could share clothing, makeup, and shoes; however, she immediately began to compare herself to all the other women: "Am I too fat? She is so much thinner than me." These thoughts soon became obsessive, and Jamie was unable to focus on her studies. She drastically cut back on what she ate and soon was consuming only 500 calories a day.

Women in sororities are at an increased risk for developing eating disorders (Zotter & Reel, 2013). One study confirmed that sorority membership may adversely affect weight outcomes, especially the disordered eating behaviors of sorority members (Averett et al., 2017). These researchers assert that sorority membership could decrease body mass index (BMI, a measure of body fat based on height and weight, used in identifying eating disorders) and contribute to certain mild disordered eating behaviors, but it is not likely they will become extreme eating-disordered behavior (Averett et al., 2017). It is not clear if sororities breed this type of behavior or women with this proclivity are drawn to such social groups. Sororities may include some women with idealized body image and who compete about weight. Jamie certainly began to compare herself unfavorably to her sorority sisters to the point that she became consumed with these thoughts. When women live together in a sorority house, they may influence one another into engaging in more risky eating behaviors.

> **Case Study**
>
> Jim had been wrestling since he was a kid. He loved the sport and was thrilled when he got a college scholarship to wrestle. The training was intense, and the coach was very demanding. The weigh-ins each week left Jim completely stressed out. Based on his weight, he would be assigned a wrestling category. He tried to eat less but found he was mentally foggy. He soon learned from some of the upper-class guys on the team how they maintained their weight. Before long, Jim was vomiting several times a day and always before weigh-ins.

Certain subpopulations of college students, including athletes and health and physical education majors, appear to be at an even higher risk for disordered eating (Zotter & Reel, 2013). Athletes involved in those sports that emphasize a player's weight—such as wrestling, swimming, and gymnastics—are at an even more increased risk than athletes in endurance or ball-game sports. College men are not immune to eating disorders. Some evidence suggests that, among men, disordered eating symptoms occurring on a regular basis remain stable over the college period (Dakanalis et al., 2016). Jim is an example of a college athlete who felt pressure to maintain his weight for wresting and soon engaged in regular vomiting. Additionally, some evidence suggests that gay and bisexual college men may show greater maladaptive eating behaviors (Matthews-Ewald et al., 2014). In a national sample of more than 65,000 college students, Lipson et al. (2019) found that 16% of transgender male and 9% of transgender female students screened positive for eating disorders, which was significantly higher than any cisgender students. Studies conducted with community samples have found that, compared with heterosexual men, gay men may be more vulnerable to eating disorders and have greater body dissatisfaction and increased bulimic and anorexic symptoms (Russell & Keel, 2002).

Researchers have also noted racial differences in eating disorders. For example, Quick and Byrd-Bredbenner (2014) found that more than other racial/ethnic groups, Black college women are more comfortable with their bodies being at higher weights and are less likely to internalize the societal message of thinness equating to beauty. In general, they displayed greater body satisfaction than other racial/ethnic groups. Those individuals who are acculturated to the Western lifestyle are also more likely to have disordered eating (Cachelin et al., 2000), as they are more likely to be influenced by social norms of thinness. Within Latinx/a/o populations, those who place a greater emphasis on the mainstream, White, dominant culture have greater body image concerns (Schooler & Lowry, 2011). The American continent tends to have a higher prevalence for all eating disorders, followed by Asia and Europe (Galmiche et al., 2019). This difference among countries may be due to genetic backgrounds, eating behaviors that may be affected by the environment, and differences in cultural factors (e.g., body image distortion influenced by the media, the multiplication of slimming diets), but also changes in lifestyle (e.g., stress, diet; Galmiche et al., 2019).

Types of Eating Disorders

The *DSM-5* recognizes several eating disorders (American Psychiatric Association [APA], 2013). The most common types observed in college students are anorexia nervosa, bulimia nervosa, and binge eating disorder. A shared trait among eating disorders is "a persistent disturbance of eating or eating-related behavior that results in the altered consumption or absorption of food and that significantly impairs physical health or psychosocial functioning" (APA, 2013, p. 329). Generally, individuals with eating disorders can display rigid eating patterns and dietary habits, and they tend to have intrusive thoughts about body weight and shape.

Anorexia Nervosa

Anorexia nervosa literally translates to "nervous loss of appetite," and a person must display all three of the following symptoms to be diagnosed with this condition. The first and primary symptom is a significantly low body weight for the individual; those who do not appear to have low body weight but have recently had significant weight loss are also considered to have this symptom. Second, the person must possess a fear of gaining weight or becoming fat that compels them to engage in behaviors that interfere with weight gain (e.g., excessive exercise, use of laxatives, skipping meals, extreme dieting). Third, the person must put enormous value on their shape and weight and/or not recognize the seriousness of the weight loss (APA, 2013). Although not a formal criterion, women may cease their menses due to the lack of body fat. Individuals with anorexia nervosa cannot recognize the inherent dangers of their condition; they are not consciously repudiating the truth (Kenny et al., 2014).

There are two main types of this disorder: one that involves weight loss efforts through dieting, fasting, or excessive exercise—and one that involves binge eating (i.e., eating more than is expected for the situation) and purging (i.e., self-induced vomiting and misuse of laxatives, enemas, or diuretics; APA, 2013). With the former type, a person fails to maintain a "healthy" body weight and may appear underweight. The person may also develop secondary symptoms such as hair loss and tooth erosion; they may have dry skin, brittle hair or nails, and a sensitivity to cold (due to extreme fat loss; Barlow et al., 2018). They may have organ failure, lose bone density, or develop a dangerous heart rhythm. This condition can be life threatening if the individual's body weight drops excessively. Individuals who binge and purge may not appear as emaciated as those who severely restrict their food intake.

APA (2013) reported that 5% of patients with anorexia nervosa die within the first 4 years of diagnosis. For those for whom the illness lasts more than 20 years, the mortality rate is 20%, with many deaths occurring suddenly (APA, 2013). Anorexia nervosa's mortality rate is related to death from starvation and metabolic collapse and suicide (Neumarker, 2000). Anorexia nervosa has a higher mortality rate than even that of depression (Papadopoulous et al., 2009). About a third of anorexia-related deaths are suicides, which is 50 times higher than occurs in the general population (Arcelus et al., 2011). Men represent 25% of individuals with anorexia nervosa, and they are at a higher risk of dying than women. This is partly due to the misconception that men don't have eating disorders, resulting in delayed diagnosis (Mond et al., 2014).

It is not uncommon for this condition to begin in young people who may be overweight. For example, someone is slightly overweight, loses some weight, and gets a lot of attention from others. This attention and new focus on the person's slimmer appearance is rewarding, so the dieting continues. Soon, the dieting is out of control, and the person is counting calories all day, every day.

Bulimia Nervosa

Bulimia nervosa is characterized by recurrent episodes of binge eating. According to the *DSM-5* (APA, 2013), an episode of binge eating must consist of both of the following: (1) eating an amount of food in a certain time period that is definitely more than what most other people would eat in the same time and in the same situation, and (2) a feeling of lack of control during this eating episode (i.e., feeling as though one cannot stop eating). The other symptom that

> **Case Study**
>
> Mark feels stressed out at college. He was top of his class in high school, but now at this prestigious college, he is just average. There are so many other smart students who seem to do well in class. His roommate is on a work-study grant, so he is not around a lot. Alone in his room, Mark often binges on candy, chips, soda, and other snacks he gets from the campus vending machines. Afterward, he feels terrible about himself and his weight. He goes to his bathroom, runs the water in the shower, and then vomits in the toilet. Despite the vomiting, Mark has found that he is still gaining weight, which only makes him feel worse about himself.

must be present is that the person engages in inappropriate compensatory behavior in order to thwart weight gain—for example, self-induced vomiting, misuse of laxatives, fasting, or excessive exercise.

In the case of Mark, he vomits shortly after his binge and does this secretly. Individuals with bulimia nervosa also largely base their self-evaluation on their body shape and weight. This condition can range from mild, where someone may engage in one to three episodes of purging or excessive exercise a week, to extreme, where an average of 14 episodes or more of inappropriate compensatory behaviors a week might take place.

Although purging is very common, it is not a particularly effective method of weight management (Fairburn, 2013). Vomiting reduces only about half of the caloric intake—and even less if the vomiting is delayed after the binge (Kaye et al., 1993). As illustrated in Mark's case, he was frustrated that his vomiting did not lead to the weight loss he desired. There are also many medical consequences from repeated vomiting. The gastric juices from the stomach can erode the enamel on teeth and harm the esophagus. The person may experience electrolyte imbalance, which can result in serious medical conditions, including effects on the heart (Barlow et al., 2018).

Those with bulimia nervosa who present for treatment are almost entirely women (90%–95%; Barlow et al., 2018). Men tend to have a later onset of the disorder and are often bisexual or gay (Matthews-Ewald et al., 2014).

Binge-Eating Disorder

Individuals with binge-eating disorder may eat more quickly than normal ("inhaling food"), eat large amounts of food even though they are not hungry, and/or eat until past the point of comfort or fullness. They may also prefer to binge eat alone so that others do not see them. After these binge episodes, they may feel guilty, disgusted with themselves, or depressed about their behavior; however, these individuals do not engage in the inappropriate compensatory behaviors such as self-induced vomiting or excessive exercise. Thus, they tend to remain at higher weights. The often-secretive nature of the bingeing means that others may not be aware of this behavior; a roommate may not even know. Like bulimia nervosa, this condition can be mild or extreme. Individuals with binge-eating disorder may binge frequently and feel distraught about this behavior, but they do not attempt to purge.

Approaching the Issue With Students

Eating disorders appear to exist on a continuum, with some behaviors frequently occurring in the population at large and other, more extreme ones happening less frequently. The skilled professional should be able to distinguish between behaviors that would not be considered pathological (e.g., overeating on occasion or typical "dieting") and those that are indicative of greater dysfunction (e.g., binge eating, dramatically restricting calories; Kenny et al., 2014).

Approaching this issue with students can be difficult, particularly because they are unlikely to come forward for help and the behaviors are often carried out in secret. Students may intentionally misreport their behavior, making assessment complicated. Professionals should be aware that individuals with eating disorders may not be honest about their symptoms, hide their behaviors, and display resistance to getting help (Abbate-Daga et al., 2013). Individuals with anorexia nervosa are often in denial; higher education professionals would be wise to not directly confront them about their behavior.

Many misconceptions and myths surround eating disorders—for example, that they occur only in wealthy White women. Higher education professionals are advised to educate themselves and examine their beliefs about disordered eating. Eating disorders do not just affect women; men and sexual minority youth appear to be at risk as well. Eating disorders can and do occur among all types of students. Further, not all eating disorders result in an observable low weight. In both bulimia nervosa and binge-eating disorder, the individual may be overweight.

Matt Zimmerman, PhD, director of training at the University of Virginia, Student Health Counseling and Psychological Services, specializes in assessing and treating eating disorders. As a member of the Student Health Eating Disorders Consult and Treatment Team, and the universitywide Coalition on Eating Disorders and Exercise Concerns, Zimmerman warns higher education professionals that "the likelihood of a good conversation the first time you approach a student with an eating disorder is low" (personal communication, March, 12, 2020). He suggests focusing on the relationship you have with the student and framing your concern around the student's level of stress. Avoid talking about or asking questions about weight, food, and eating, as the student is not likely to respond well. The recommended approach is to frame the issue as a problem with stress. The notion of stress is more palatable for those with eating disorders. Saying something like, "You looked stressed. Maybe classes are taking a toll on you physically and mentally. It might help to get some support" or "You look fatigued and at your limit." Stress is not uncommon among these students. For many, the combination of leaving home, difficult course work, living independent from parents, and managing a new social atmosphere is contributing to their stress and may be fueling the disordered eating.

The National Eating Disorders Collaboration (n.d.) advises using "I statements" when expressing concerns to a student suspected of having an eating disorder—"I am concerned" or "It makes me scared for you"—instead of "You statements," such as "You need to stop this diet" or "You look terrible," which can make people feel guilty or defensive. Be patient and understanding. Listen to the student's story without judgment. Try not to get frustrated; the person is not doing this intentionally to upset you. Remember that the student in front of you may be very worried about gaining weight, even if they look very thin to you. This body dysmorphia is often very difficult for untrained professionals to comprehend, but it is an essential feature of some conditions.

There is a tremendous amount of shame with eating disorders. If you directly ask about eating patterns, you are likely to get a kind, polite response—and the student may avoid you from then on. When a student with an eating disorder is approached about it directly, they now feel threatened and fear that their coping skill may be taken away. The person who is closest to the student may be the best choice of who should approach them, but remember that the focus should remain on the student's overall well-being and not their eating or exercising habits.

It is unlikely that a student will spontaneously disclose an eating disorder to a professional. Individuals with anorexia nervosa seldom seek treatment on their own (Barlow et al., 2018) and are more likely to be pressured into treatment by a family member (Fairburn & Cooper, 2014). Those in treatment are not coming voluntarily and have likely been referred by someone who is exerting leverage on them—a parent, friend, roommate, or partner. So, if the student is complaining that everyone is bugging them about their weight, a good response might be, "That must be so frustrating to constantly hear that." The goal should be to help the student feel understood. For students living on campus, the family may not be aware of the extreme weight loss. It is more probable that, as a professional, you may be alerted to extreme weight loss or observe behaviors that are alarming. Friends or roommates of the student may also come to you worried about their friend and unsure of what to do to help.

When approaching someone about an eating disorder, express your worries in a caring, nonconfrontational way. Arrange when you can speak privately with the student. Remain calm, focused, positive, and respectful during the conversation. It is important to be nonjudgmental. Do not offer advice about eating. Do not push students to disclose more than they want to during the meeting. One of the difficulties faced by students with disordered eating is that they cannot just *avoid* eating. Students who have problems with drugs or alcohol can be encouraged and supported in their abstinence; this is not the case with food.

Understand that people who suffer from eating disorders often experience shame and embarrassment, which contributes to their lack of disclosure about their behavior (Berg & Peterson, 2013). Using nonspecific counseling techniques such as empathy, unconditional positive regard, and reflection will increase rapport with the student and may encourage them to reveal symptoms. What may be difficult to understand is that individuals with anorexia nervosa may be proud of their restrictive self-control. It is not uncommon to find several people with this condition compare (or compete) for who has eaten the fewest calories per day. At the same time, these individuals are never satisfied with their weight loss—thus the resulting emaciated look that is concerning to everyone except the person with anorexia nervosa. Also, statements such as "You look healthy to me" can be misinterpreted by students to think they look fat, so avoid making comments about the student's weight.

Nearly half of individuals who report severe impairment due to their eating disorder receive treatment for their condition, and less than

20% with severe impairment seek such treatment from a mental health professional (Mond et al., 2007). This impairment can take the form of difficulty concentrating on school work, social isolation or withdrawal, and depressed mood. Research has shown that the combination of perfectionistic tendencies with emotion dysregulation may be a key to understanding which individuals at high risk for or with eating disorders may experience the highest levels of clinical impairment (Byrne et al., 2016). In men, the psychological factors that underlie the initiation of recurrent behavioral symptoms of eating disorders are the same as those that contribute to the persistence of eating disorders: negative affectivity, body dissatisfaction, self-objectification, and lower self-esteem (Dakanalis et al., 2016). In the case of eating disorders, without professional intervention, symptoms may worsen, resulting in adverse consequences and impaired functioning (Wilfley et al., 2013). If you encounter someone who has struggled with an eating disorder, remember you don't need to fully understand the condition; just be there and be present and ready to help.

The appendix of this book provides some reputable online sources that can help students with eating disorders; however, many websites are dangerous and promote unhealthy habits. Sites referred to as "pro-ana" (pro-anorexia), "pro-mia" (pro-bulimia), or "thinspo" can contain pictures of emaciated bodies and include tips on how to starve oneself. If a student tells you that they are getting help online, be sure to ask about what sites and social media they are accessing.

When and How to Make a Referral to Counseling

The best advice for professionals when they encounter a student with *any* suspected eating disorder is to refer the student. It would be prudent to determine if your campus health center has an eating disorder specialist or a task force that deals with eating disorders. Some universities have integrated multidisciplinary teams to handle cases of eating disorders. They consist of professionals from medicine, women's health, psychiatry, psychology, and nutrition. While such teams may not be equipped to treat all cases, depending on severity or the model of the center, they can typically consult on a case or assess and recommend higher levels of care than are available on campus. Students are more likely to accept a referral to a medical professional than a mental health professional. As mentioned previously, anorexia nervosa can be life threatening if the individual maintains an unhealthy weight, is emaciated, and remains medically unstable due to the severity of the eating disorder. Bulimia nervosa can also be very dangerous, due to risks caused by electrolyte imbalances (disrupted sodium and potassium levels), which can lead to renal failure and disrupted heartbeat; this condition doesn't always allow you to "see" how sick or at risk someone may be, but the medical consequences can be severe. Medical professionals can determine the severity of the condition and order appropriate blood work. Blood screenings can examine electrolytes and other functions that are typically not performed by regular physicians. Mem Wood, clinical director at Veritas Collaborative's Adult Hospital in Durham, North Carolina, advises that the important message is that treatment and management from professionals who specialize in eating disorders is essential (e.g., therapist, nutritionist, physician). There can be severe consequences for individuals who attempt to "recover" on their own—for example, by rapidly increasing their level of food intake.

There are multiple levels of care for the person with an eating disorder, and professionals trained in assessment are the best to determine the level. If the student's weight is severely underweight or purging is frequent, or they are severely restricting their fluid intake, referral to an inpatient unit would be recommended. Once stabilization is achieved and maintained, the patient can transition to a lower level of care for further treatment. Outpatient treatment, consisting of weekly or twice weekly individual and group sessions, may be appropriate for some students. Professionals should be aware of local eating disorder treatment centers in order to make an appropriate referral.

Although the instinct for a higher education professional would be to refer a student with an eating disorder concern to the college counseling center, it may not be the best course of action. Counseling centers are often understaffed and overburdened. The Center for Collegiate Mental Health (2021) found that in the academic year 2020–2021, the average client per counselor case load at college counseling centers was 90 students. In fact, it is estimated that less than 20% of college students who screen positive for eating disorders receive treatment (Eisenberg et al., 2011). The student with an eating disorder may be worried about dropping out of school for treatment. One way higher education professionals can assist with this concern is to explore the options or possibilities for the student to remain enrolled (e.g., distance learning/online classes, medical leave) and provide support for this very real concern.

Some research suggests a high rate of suicidality in college students with eating disorders, making this a condition of greatest concern. Eating disorder symptoms, even at below clinical levels, were highly predictive of suicidality in a recent sample of more than 70,000 college students (Lipson & Sonneville, 2020). Compared with students with no apparent eating disorder symptoms, students with the highest symptom levels had 11 times higher odds of attempting suicide (Lipson & Sonneville, 2020). If there is any indication that a student is suicidal, an assessment should be made, the student's parents should be contacted, and the student should be referred for immediate psychiatric help.

Conclusion

Eating habits can range among college students as they adjust to a new schedule, eating on campus, and exposure to different foods. The stress of college life can cause some students to overeat, while others lose weight due to skipping meals. Although some variation is expected, students who are displaying drastic changes in weight and eating habits should be of concern to higher education professionals. Some students may also come to college with preexisting eating disorders that are exacerbated at school. The hidden nature of these conditions as well as the denial and shame frequently felt by these students will often cause them to not ask for help. The role of the higher education professional is to be aware of the signs and symptoms and be able to nonjudgmentally approach students who seem to be suffering. Given the potentially fatal outcome for some of these conditions, severely maladaptive eating patterns must be approached with students in a caring and compassionate manner. There is a range of educational and treatment options, and connecting students with the right one is critical to their recovery.

References

Abbate-Daga, G., Amianto, F., Delsedime, N., De-Bacco, C., & Fassino, S. (2013). Resistance to treatment and change in anorexia nervosa: A clinical overview. *BMC Psychiatry, 13*, 294–311. http://doi.org/10.1186/1471-244X-13-294

American College Health Association. (2022). *American College Health Association–National College Health Assessment III: Undergraduate student reference group executive summary fall 2021.* https://www.acha.org/documents/ncha/NCHA-III_FALL_2021_UNDERGRADUATE_REFERENCE_GROUP_EXECUTIVE_SUMMARY.pdf

American Psychiatric Association. (2013). *Diagnostic and statistical manual of mental disorders* (5th ed.).

Arcelus, J., Mitchell, A. J., Wales, J., & Nielsen, S. (2011). Mortality rates in patients with anorexia nervosa and other eating disorders: A meta-analysis of 36 studies. *Archives of General Psychiatry, 68*(7), 724–731. https://doi.org/10.1001/archgenpsychiatry.2011.74

Averett, S., Terrizzi, S., & Wang, Y. (2017). The effect of sorority membership on eating disorders, body weight, and disordered-eating behaviors. *Health Economics, 26*(7), 875–891. https://doi.org/10.1002/hec.3360

Barlow, D., Durand, M., & Hofmann, S. (2018). *Abnormal psychology: An integrative approach* (8th ed.). Cengage Learning.

Berg, K. C., & Peterson, C. B. (2013). Assessment and diagnosis of eating disorders. In L. H. Choate (Ed.), *Eating disorders and obesity: A counselor's guide to prevention and treatment* (pp. 91–117). American Counseling Association.

Byrne, M. E., Eichen, D. M., Fitzsimmons-Craft, E., Taylor, C. B., & Wilfley, D. E. (2016). Perfectionism, emotion dysregulation, and affective disturbance in relation to clinical impairment in college-age women at high risk for or with eating disorders. *Eating Behaviors, 23*, 131–136. https://doi.org/10.1016/j.eatbeh.2016.09.004

Cachelin, F. M., Veisel, C., Barzegarnazari, E., & Striegel-Moore, R. H. (2000). Disordered eating, acculturation, and treatment-seeking in a community sample of Hispanic, Asian, black, and white women. *Psychology of Women Quarterly, 24*(3), 244–233. https://doi.org/10.1111/j.1471-6402.2000.tb00206.x

Carithers-Thomas, J. A., Bradford, S. H., Keshock, C. M., & Pugh, S. F. (2010). Freshman fifteen: Fact or fiction? *College Student Journal, 44*(2), 419–424.

Center for Collegiate Mental Health. (2021). Clinical load index, 2020-2021 distribution. https://ccmh.shinyapps.io/CLI-app/_w_be1991b3/Clinical%20Load%20Index%20(CLI)%20Guide.pdf

Dakanalis, A., Clerici, M., Caslini, M., Gaudio, S., Serino, S., Riva, G., & Carrà, G. (2016). Predictors of initiation and persistence of recurrent binge eating and inappropriate weight compensatory behaviors in college men. *International Journal of Eating Disorders, 49*(6), 581–590. https://doi.org/10.1002/eat.22535

Derenne, J., & Beresin, E. (2018). Body image, media, and eating disorders—a 10-year update. *Academic Psychiatry, 42*, 129–134. https://doi.org/10.1007/s40596-017-0832-z

Eisenberg, D., Nicklett, E. J., Roeder, K., & Kirz, N. E. (2011). Eating disorder symptoms among college students: Prevalence, persistence, correlates, and treatment-seeking. *Journal of American College Health, 59*(8), 700–707. https://doi.org/10.1080/07448481.2010.546461

Fairburn, C. G. (2013). *Overcoming binge eating* (2nd ed.). Guilford Press.

Fairburn, C. G., & Cooper, Z. (2014). Eating disorders: A transdiagnostic protocol. In D. H. Barlow (Ed.), *Clinical handbook of psychological disorders: A step-by-step treatment manual* (5th ed., pp. 670–702). Guilford Press.

Franko, D. L., Mintz, L. B., Villapiano, M., Green, T. C., Mainelli, D., Folensbee, L., Butler, S. F., Davidson, M. M., Hamilton, E., Little, D., Kearns, M., & Budman, S. H. (2005). Food, mood and attitude: Reducing risk for eating disorders in college women. *Health Psychology, 24*(6), 567–578. https://doi.org/10.1037/0278-6133.24.6.567

Galmiche, M., Déchelotte, P., Lambert, G., Tavolacci, P. M. (2019). Prevalence of eating disorders over the 2000–2018 period: A systematic literature review, *The American Journal of Clinical Nutrition, 109*(5), 1402–1413. https://doi.org/10.1093/ajcn/nqy342

Golden, N. H., Schneider, M., Wood, C., & American Academy of Pediatrics Committee on Nutrition. (2016). Preventing obesity and eating disorders in adolescents. *Pediatrics, 138*(3), e1–e16. https://doi.org/10.1542/peds.2016-1649

Hoffman, D. J., Policastro, P., Quick, V., & Lee, S. (2006). Changes in body weight and fat mass of men and women in the first year of college: A study of the "freshman 15." *Journal of American College Health, 55*(1), 41–46. https://doi.org/10.3200/jach.55.1.41-46

Hudson, J., Hiripi, E., Pope, H., & Kessler, R. (2007). The prevalence and correlates of eating disorders in the national comorbidity survey replication. *Biological Psychiatry, 61*(3), 348–358. https://dx.doi.org/10.1016%2Fj.biopsych.2006.03.040

Kaye, W. H., Weltzin, T. E., Hsu, L. G., McConaha, C. W., & Bolton, B. (1993). Amount of calories retained after binge eating and vomiting. *The American Journal of Psychiatry, 150*(6), 969–971. https://doi.org/10.1176/ajp.150.6.969

Kenny, M. C., Ward-Lichterman, M., & Abdelmonem, M. H. (2014). The expansion and clarification of feeding and eating disorders in the *DSM-5*. *The Professional Counselor, 4*(3), 246–256. https://tpcjournal.nbcc.org/the-expansion-and-clarification-of-feeding-and-eating-disorders-in-the-dsm-5

Lebow, J., Sim, L., & Kransdorf, L. (2015). Prevalence of a history of overweight and obesity in adolescents with restrictive eating disorders. *Journal of Adolescent Health, 56*(1), 19–24. http://dx.doi.org/10.1016/j.jadohealth.2014.06.005

Lipson, S. K., Raifman, J., Abelson, S., & Reisner, S. L. (2019). Gender minority mental health in the U.S.: Results of a national survey on college campuses. *American Journal of Preventive Medicine, 57*(3), 293–301. https://doi.org/10.1016/j.amepre.2019.04.025

Lipson, S. K., & Sonneville, K. R. (2020). Understanding suicide risk and eating disorders in college student populations: Results from a national study. *International Journal of Eating Disorders, 53*(2), 229–238. https://doi.org/10.1002/eat.23188

Matthews-Ewald, M., Zullig, K. J., & Ward, R. M. (2014). Sexual orientation and disordered eating behaviors among self-identified male and female college students. *Eating Behaviors, 15*(3), 441–444. https://doi.org/10.1016/j.eatbeh.2014.05.002

Mond, J. M., Hay, P. J., Rodgers, B., & Owen, C. (2007). Recurrent binge eating with and without the "undue influence of weight or shape on self-evaluation": Implications for the diagnosis of binge eating disorder. *Behaviour Research and Therapy, 45*(5), 929–938. https://doi.org/10.1016/j.brat.2006.08.011

Mond, J., Mitchison, D., & Hay, P. (2014). Eating disordered behavior in men: Prevalence, impairment in quality of life, and implications for prevention and health promotion. In L. Cohn & R. Lemberg (Eds.), *Current findings on males with eating disorders* (pp. 195–215). Routledge.

National Eating Disorders Collaboration. (n.d.). *What to say and do*. https://nedc.com.au/support-and-services/supporting-someone/what-to-say-and-do

Neumarker, K.-J. (2000). Mortality rates and causes of death. *European Eating Disorders Review, 8,* 181–187. https://doi.org/10.1002/(SICI)1099-0968(200003)8:2<181::AID-ERV336>3.0.CO;2-%23

Papadopoulos, F. C., Ekbom, A., Brandt, L., & Ekselius, L. (2009). Excess mortality, causes of death and prognostic factors in anorexia nervosa. *The British Journal of Psychiatry, 194*(1), 10–17. https://doi.org/10.1192/bjp.bp.108.054742

Quick, V. M., & Byrd-Bredbenner, C. (2014). Disordered eating, socio-cultural media influencers, body image, and psychological factors among a racially/ethnically diverse population of college women. *Eating Behaviors, 15*(1), 37–41. https://doi.org/10.1016/j.eatbeh.2013.10.005

Rohde, P., Stice, E., Shaw, H., Gau, J. M., & Ohls, O. C. (2017). Age effects in eating disorder baseline risk factors and prevention intervention effects. *International Journal of Eating Disorders, 50*(11), 1273–1280. https://doi.org/10.1002/eat.22775

Russell, C. J., & Keel, P. K. (2002). Homosexuality as a specific risk factor for eating disorders in men. *International Journal of Eating Disorders, 31*(3), 300–306. https://doi.org/10.1002/eat.10036

Schooler, D., & Lowry, L. S. (2011). Hispanic/Latino body images. In T. F. Cash & L. Smolak (Eds.), *Body image: A handbook of science, practice, and prevention* (2nd ed., pp. 237–243). Guilford Press.

Schwitzer, A. M., Bergholz, K., Dore, T., & Salimi, L. (1998). Eating disorders among college women: Prevention, education, and treatment responses. *Journal of American College Health, 46*(5), 199–207. https://doi.org/10.1080/07448489809600223

Stice, E., Marti, C. N., & Rohde, P. (2013). Prevalence, incidence, impairment, and course of the proposed *DSM-5* eating disorder diagnoses in an 8-year prospective community study of young women. *Journal of Abnormal Psychology, 122*(2), 445–457. https://doi.org/10.1037/a0030679

Wilfley, D. E., Agras, W. S., & Taylor, C. B. (2013). Reducing the burden of eating disorders: A model for population-based prevention and treatment for university and college campuses. *International Journal of Eating Disorders, 46*(5), 529–532. https://dx.doi.org/10.1002%2Feat.22117

Zotter, D., & Reel, J. (2013). Effective prevention programs in college and university settings. In L. H. Choate (Ed.), *Eating disorders and obesity: A counselor's guide to prevention and treatment* (pp. 241–263). American Counseling Association. https://doi.org/10.1002/9781119221708.ch11

CHAPTER 10

Sexual Assault and Victimization

Many students arrive at college with a history of sexual abuse, while others may be victimized while enrolled in college. Understanding the consequences of sexual assault for students is important in helping them recover. Higher education professionals need to be knowledgeable and sensitive to the emotional and behavioral issues that may arise as a result of acquaintance rape or sexual assault. Although many colleges and universities have campaigns against sexual assault, it remains prevalent. Victims suffer from fears of sexually transmitted infections and pregnancy. Long-term effects can include depression, anxiety, and posttraumatic stress disorder. While this crime often goes unreported, higher education professionals need to be astute to the signs of trauma responses in order to best help victims recover. Approaching this topic with students requires compassion and care.

Basic Signs and Symptoms of Sexual Assault

Sexual assault is an unfortunately all too common experience for college students. It has reached such epic proportions that the U.S. government has addressed it through legislation. Most recently, former President Barack Obama launched the "It's On Us" (that is, it's on us to stop sexual assault) campaign in 2014, which was a social-media-driven effort to raise awareness of sexual assault on college campuses. This campaign led to increased prevention and education programming for all students on campus as well as improved responses of college administrators to allegations. The film *The Hunting Ground* (Dick, 2015) is a documentary about the incidence of sexual assault on college campuses in the United States and the apparent failure of college administrators to deal with it adequately. In the wake of the #MeToo movement, there is increased attention on sexual violence against women across the globe.

Although anyone can be a victim of sexual assault on campus, women constitute the majority of victims.[1] One study found that approximately 20% of women experienced sexual assault while in college (Krebs et al., 2007). College-aged women (18 to 24 years) are more likely to be sexually assaulted than women of any other age group (Sinozich & Langton, 2014). A more recent study of 27 U.S. college campuses estimated that 26% of undergraduate women and 6% of undergraduate men are victims of sexual assault (Cantor et al., 2015). A systematic review that examined research conducted on college sexual assault between the years 2000 to 2015 found that unwanted sexual contact, including sexual coercion, was most

---

[1] The term *victim* is used throughout this chapter. The authors are aware of the use of the term *survivor* for those who have survived sexual assault and agree with the empowering nature of this word. However, given that we are focusing primarily on working with a student following an assault, we believe the term *victim* is more applicable.

prevalent on college campuses, followed by drug- or alcohol-facilitated rape, and third, forcible rape both attempted or completed (Fedina et al., 2016). Although sexual assault can occur at any time during college, the first year is reported to be a very high-risk time for female sexual assault (Humphrey & White, 2000). For example, the national Sexual Victimization of College Women study that surveyed 4,446 college women found that almost 9% of the women experienced unwanted sexual contact within an academic year, and nearly 3% experienced rape (Fisher et al., 2000). Being a sexual minority also puts one at risk for sexual victimization. Coulter et al. (2017) found that while cisgender heterosexual women are at high risk for sexual assault, transgender people and cisgender bisexual women have even higher odds of sexual assault. Ford and Soto-Marquez (2016) found that bisexual women report the highest rates of sexual assault by their senior year (38%), and lesbian women report the lowest rates of any group (11%). Gay men (24%) and bisexual men (18%) experience high rates of sexual assault by their senior year, both markedly higher than rates of heterosexual men (Ford & Soto-Marquez, 2016). Further, 21% of college students who identify as transgender, genderqueer, and gender nonconforming have experienced sexual assault (Rape, Abuse, & Incest National Network [RAINN], 2021).

Aside from gender and sexual orientation, other factors put one at risk of sexual assault. The "hookup culture," where casual sexual activity without emotional connections or relationship commitments is also believed to be associated with the rise in sexual assaults across college campuses (Allison & Risman, 2013; England et al., 2007). Ford and Soto-Marquez (2016) found that college victims of sexual assault tended to be more engaged in hooking up, which has been loosely associated with the college party scene. Higher education professionals should keep in mind that traditional-aged college students are still developing and forging their identities. Many students may be away from home for the first time and surrounded by same-age peers who may be engaging in risky behaviors, which may result in them doing the same. Past sexual victimization has also been found to be a strong predictor of subsequent assault (Roodman & Clum, 2001). In Turchik et al.'s (2010) study, the strongest predictor of sexual assault over the academic quarter (8 weeks) was the report of previous sexual victimization since the age of 14.

> ### Case Study
>
> John met Kyle in his Introduction to Sociology class. They sat next to each other during every class and often talked before or after class. John thought Kyle was cute, so when Kyle asked him to go out, he was thrilled. They exchanged phone numbers, and Kyle texted John to tell him about a party at a friend's off-campus apartment. John told his roommates, and they excitedly talked about the "big date." John met Kyle outside the school's library, and they walked together to the party. The music was loud and the party was crowded but they had fun dancing and talking. They both were drinking, and while John felt a "buzz," he was not drunk. Kyle offered to walk him home after the party. John was excited as they had gotten along well all night. He invited Kyle into his room, and they began to kiss. As things got more heated, John told Kyle to stop, but he would not. Kyle put his hand over John's mouth and raped him. John was in shock when Kyle got dressed to leave. John confronted Kyle about what he did, and he said, "What did you think would happen when you invited me back to your room?"
>
> In the morning, John's roommates asked him how the date went. He told them it was fine. He could not find the words to tell them what happened. He was embarrassed, ashamed, and afraid they would blame him. John never went to the campus clinic or told anyone. He still saw Kyle in class but he did not speak to him. Sometimes at night, John would flash back in his mind to how he was raped. He would have trouble sleeping or wake up and feel as though Kyle were in his

> room. He tried to act as though nothing happened, but he felt sad and confused. A few weeks later, midterms were mounting, and he was unable to concentrate on studying. After a few days of lying in bed, one of John's roommates entered his room and found John unshaven and looking terrible. It was only then, pushed by his roommate, that John finally disclosed what happened.

Alcohol seems to exacerbate rates of sexual assault: 50% to 70% of incidents involve alcohol use (Abbey et al., 2004; Reed et al., 2009). The use of alcohol and drugs can influence sexual assault in several complex ways. Overuse of alcohol and drugs can lead women and men to be unable to provide consent for sexual activity, or they may be given a drug to render them incapacitated (often referred to as date rape drugs). Krebs et al. (2009) found that most sexual assaults occurred when women voluntarily consumed alcohol, but a few occurred when women were given a drug without their knowledge or consent. When women are intoxicated, they are less likely to report the assault to the police, more likely to blame themselves, and more likely to be blamed by others for the rape (Orchowski et al., 2013). Men may also not be able to fend off their attackers, especially in cases involving incapacitating substances (Bateman & Wathen, 2015). Men can be rendered confused, disoriented, or even unconscious when drugs such as Rohypnol (Roofies) or large amounts of alcohol are involved. As John's case showed, both he and Kyle had been drinking. He did not report the assault to the police or anyone else, fearing the response and believing Kyle's blame of him. John had just met Kyle, but sexual assault can also happen within the context of a longer-term relationship. In fact, most sexual assaults of women are perpetrated by someone known to the victim, including a current partner. This is also true for men, where more than half (52%) reported being raped by an acquaintance (Black et al. 2011). Acquaintance rape (where the perpetrator is known to the victim, either recently known or a partner

> **Case Study**
>
> Jane and Ethan had been dating for a few months. He was a fun guy, and she enjoyed hanging out with him. One night, after they left a social gathering, they went back to her apartment. Jane remembers saying she did not want to have sex. Ethan ignored her protests and kept pushing her. Despite her resistance, Ethan had sex with her. Jane was stunned and could not believe her boyfriend would do this. She thought rapes only happened with someone you didn't know while walking alone on a dark street. She left his apartment quickly without speaking to him. Ethan called and texted her, but she did not reply. He apologized and did not understand why she was so upset. He said, "We've had sex before. What's the big deal?" When her friends asked why she was not dating Ethan anymore, she just said they had differences they could not resolve. She never told anyone about that night.

or spouse) is more common than stranger rape; the most prevalent perpetrator is a current partner (Persson et al., 2018).

Students who have suffered an intense traumatic experience, no matter what kind, experience a range of reactions. Victims of sexual violence can display signs of depression, anxiety, and posttraumatic stress disorder (PTSD; Kirkpatrick et al., 2007; Nickerson et al., 2013). They may feel socially isolated, sad, suspicious, angry, and powerless (Bollinger et al., 2018; Ottens & Hotelling, 2001; Ullman et al., 2007). Victims of sexual assault may experience relationship difficulties as well as engage in risky behaviors. They are also more likely to abuse drugs and alcohol and to drop out of school compared to students who have never experienced sexual violence (Gidycz et al., 2008; Zinzow et al., 2011). It is not uncommon for a victim to experience intense feelings of shame and guilt following a sexual assault. The victim may also feel down or sad and have difficulty getting out of bed or attending classes. The victim may also experience trouble concentrating in class and begin to fall behind on their studies. Some of these symptoms are illustrated in the case of John after his rape. While these are all signs of depression, they are also "normal" reactions to a sexual trauma. Anxiety may also increase in some victims. They may be hypervigilant, have an increased startle response ("jumping" when hearing a loud noise), or seem "on edge." Some victims can return to "normal functioning" within a few months after experiencing a traumatic event, but for others, the trauma may stay with them and disrupt their everyday activities. While many victims may suffer from these conditions, it is important to note the strength of survivors, encourage relational resiliency, and understand that not all victims will experience PTSD or other mental health disorders (Bryant-Davis et al., 2011).

While the effects on the victim can be debilitating, friends who learn about a friend's sexual assault can also experience negative emotional reactions. Friends of sexual assault victims who were told about the assault afterward report feelings of anger and emotional distress; physically witnessing the assault can be even more traumatic (Ahrens & Campbell, 2000; Banyard et al., 2010). Thus, students who may be present when another student is raped, as can happen in fraternity houses for example, can also experience distress.

The most severe reaction to a traumatic event is PTSD. This occurs when a person is exposed to or directly experiences or learns about a traumatic event, such as sexual violence, serious injury, or death (or threatened death). A student who is the victim of sexual assault or learns about a friend's sexual assault might meet this criteria for PTSD. While the criteria for a professional diagnosis of PTSD are beyond the scope of this chapter, the higher education professional should be aware of common signs. Some victims, like John, will have flashbacks where they feel as though they are back in the situation. Others will have dreams about the traumatic event and will avoid thoughts, feelings, or reminders about it, (e.g., a student who does not want to attend college parties because she was sexually assaulted after one). Some victims have difficulty recalling aspects of the trauma, which may lead others around them to erroneously think the trauma did not occur. For example, if a rape victim tells their friend they cannot remember what room they were in when they were raped or exactly what time of the night it was, their friend may question the validity of the claim. However, it is well established that memory during traumatic events can be disrupted (Brewin, 2007). Hardy et al. (2009) contended that commonly occurring psychological reactions to trauma may affect victims' ability to recollect and talk about sexual assault. This may also ultimately affect their willingness to report to authorities. Victims may also blame themselves for the trauma, lose interest in activities that usually give them pleasure, and not be able to feel good or happy about anything. People who develop this condition after a traumatic event may show symptoms immediately or can have a delayed reaction of up to 3 months after the traumatic event. Victims of sexual assault may show signs of PTSD but not meet the full criteria, but the level of distress they experience can still be debilitating. Women are more likely than men to have this condition, but this is believed to be related to the fact that more women are victims of sexual assault (American Psychiatric Association, 2013). PTSD is also associated with an increased risk of suicide (Wilcox et al., 2009). Students who have PTSD and have suffered a traumatic event are more likely to attempt suicide than those who have suffered a traumatic event and have not developed PTSD (Wilcox et al., 2009). Students who are suffering from PTSD can have serious impairment and may not be able to function properly at school.

Approaching the Issue With Students

Sexual assaults on campus are underreported (Paul et al., 2013; Sabina & Ho, 2014), even though many students believe it is important to report them. Most rapes and attempted rapes (between 63%

and 74%) are not reported to the police (Rennison & Dodge, 2012). Reasons include knowing the offender well, believing the assault to be a personal matter, fear of reprisal, and believing the police are biased against victims. Sexual, gender, and racial/ethnic minorities may be mistrustful, or discriminated against, which may also affect their rates of reporting sexual assault (Boulware et al., 2003; Frankowski, 2004; Grant et al., 2011). Research has found that sexual assault survivors are likely to disclose to a friend (Banyard et al., 2010). It is possible that the friend may approach or seek help from a higher education professional. In these cases, it would be wise to encourage the friend to come with the victim to your office so that as the higher education professional you can provide assistance.

If a student does disclose sexual assault to you, it is critical that you respond in an appropriately supportive manner. When speaking with a victim, focus on listening and supporting, rather than encouraging the victim to report to the authorities. There are several reasons to not push a victim to report to law enforcement, including that the response from law enforcement may not always be helpful to the victim and some victims end up feeling revictimized. You should provide empathic statements as victims share their story, such as, "That must have been frightening" or "Of course you had no idea that would happen on the date." You may also gently support victims for sharing their story with you, with statements such as, "I am sorry that happened to you, but I am glad you feel comfortable enough to tell me" or "I can see how hard it is for you to tell me about that night. Thank you for sharing with me." Never blame the victim or question their judgment about the situation—that is, *never* say, "Well you did go home with him" or "Sounds like you changed your mind at some point about having sex. So he was probably confused." These statements blame the victim and will only lead to greater distress. You should also not question why the student did or did not disclose the assault at the time it occurred. There are many reasons victims do not come forward, including self-blame, fear of being blamed by others, fear they will not be believed, or fear of retaliation by the perpetrator, and sometimes they are too traumatized to go to authorities (Engel, 2008). Research has found that the reaction to a disclosure can influence the development of symptoms for the victim, with a negative social reaction more likely to lead to higher levels of PTSD symptoms (Ullman & Filipas, 2001; Ullman et al., 2007).

A clear message to convey to all victims, no matter their age or sexual orientation, is that the perpetrators are always to blame for sexual violence. While the victim may want to talk about the perpetrator, try to keep the focus on the victim's feelings. For example, the higher education professional who is talking with John can say, "I hear what you think about Kyle, but I am mostly concerned with how you feel and how this is affecting you." Do not make threats against the offender, such as, "Kyle will pay for this." This advice also applies to making promises about events you cannot control. For example, you do not know what the outcome of a legal investigation might be, so don't promise that the offender will be punished. Promise only what you know you can deliver, such as, "I'll be here for you while you handle this situation, and I will make sure we get you the services you need right now." While you will want to keep the information a victim shares confidential, higher education professionals may have a responsibility to report cases to administration via the Clery Act (see Chapter 3).

As a supportive listener, you do not need to ask for details of what happened. If the victim wishes to share details with you, you can listen. However, it is important not to push a victim to talk about aspects of the sexual assault if they are not ready or able. Understand that it is difficult to talk about such acts or abuse to a stranger while experiencing feelings of self-blame or shock. You do not want to appear voyeuristic or appear to be seeking gratuitous details. While "breaking the silence" can be helpful, it is important to let victims share what they feel comfortable sharing, when they feel comfortable sharing it. You do not need to know the details in order to provide support.

Remain calm when victims share their story with you. You may be upset or outraged by what you hear, but getting upset will not help the victim. Allow the victim to express a range of emotions regarding what happened. Understand that the victim may be confused and sorting out how they feel. The victim may feel a range of emotions, such as shock, denial, and/or anger. Be patient as the victim reveals the situation. At times the victim may want to remain silent; stay focused on the victim and use appropriate, attentive body language, but do not push for disclosure. If you find yourself sitting in silence with the victim, you can say, "I'm here if you want to talk or don't want to talk." Saying this in a calm, reassuring manner will help the victim feel more in control of the situation.

Have tissues accessible because the victim may cry. Since the victim lost control during the assault, let them make as many decisions as possible about what their next steps will be. Ask them, "Is there someone you want to call?" or "What do you want to do now?" And then provide some options. It is important to normalize the feelings that a victim is having. For example, some victims report feeling numb and not being able to experience any feelings. You might say, "I think the way you feel is fairly common. It's understandable that you would feel frightened or scared." Avoid comparing their situation to that of another student. Each person handles their experience differently. Don't say, "Well at least you had only one rapist. I had another student who was raped by two men." This is not going to help the victim; instead, it takes the focus off the victim and sounds like you are minimizing the experience.

Table 10.1

What to Do and Not Do With a Victim of Sexual Assault

Do	Don't
Listen calmly to the victim	Question the victim's judgment
Support and believe the victim	Blame the victim for any action they took
Keep what the victim tells you confidential	Push the victim to make a police report
Offer resources on and off campus	Tell the victim to move on from the assault
Give the victim choices	Tell the victim you know how they feel
	Compare to other victims' experiences

There is a tendency in our general culture to view the victim as at fault. Higher education professionals need to examine their beliefs regarding rape and sexual assault and gain education on this form of victimization. Since many others may respond in an unsupportive manner to a victim who was drinking at the time of the assault, it falls to the higher education professional to provide a supportive, nonjudgmental, and accepting attitude toward the victim. Research has shown that when the victim had been drinking before the sexual assault, people provide less emotional support and assign greater victim responsibility and lower perpetrator responsibility for the assault (Untied et al., 2012). Table 10.1 provides examples of recommended ways to respond.

It is important to keep in mind that how women label a sexual assault should not be used to determine whether victimization occurred (Fisher et al., 2003). Many women will not label sexual assault as such (Orchowski et al., 2013). Men, too, may not consider a rape to have occurred if they have been forced into sexual contact (Weare, 2018). Most women who reported experiences of sexual victimization did not see themselves as victims, and 38% labeled their sexual victimization as a serious miscommunication (Orchowski et al., 2013). When the victim knew the perpetrator (acquaintance) and/or they were using substances at the time of the assault, the victim was again more likely to label the sexual assault as a serious miscommunication. There are other reasons victims may not acknowledge that a rape occurred, including that it does not fit the "stereotype" of a forced sexual act by a stranger, desire to minimize the experience, or fear of the stigma of being labeled a victim. One role of the higher education professional may be to educate the victim about what happened. For example, "Sam, what you are telling me is that your date forced you to have sex with him. While you may not see it that way now, that is considered rape" or "I know it may be hard for you to think of yourself as having been raped, but I want you to know that is what happened to you; it is not OK and it is not your fault."

When and How to Make a Referral to Counseling

When the trauma seems to affect a student's daily functioning, it may be best to refer them for professional counseling. Some signs of this would include not going to classes, poor hygiene (i.e., not showering, wearing the same clothes without washing), and reports of depressed mood that interferes with the student's ability to carry out everyday tasks. Another time to refer might be when the student is displaying signs of PTSD, given the risk of suicide. In your role as a higher education professional, you might say, "Pat, I know this has been hard on you. I am worried that you are falling behind in class and don't seem to be able to cope with some of your everyday demands. While I am happy to talk to you, I wonder if we might think about talking to someone else—a professional with more training to help you." Another approach might be, "It seems as though you are really struggling since that night. I am worried about how depressed you are, and I want to try and help you feel better. Would you consider talking to someone else about how you feel?"

Another instance that may warrant referral for counseling is when the student reports a history of sexual victimization. Higher education professionals who encounter students who have been sexually assaulted should be aware that the current sexual assault may not be their first or most severe assault (Carey et al., 2015; Martin et al., 2011). A history of sexual assault is a risk factor for subsequent assault, so students who come forward with sexual assaults on campus may also be dealing with other past victimizations. Read et al. (2011) found that 7% of incoming freshmen in their study reported previous sexual assault (11% of women; 2% of men). Having experienced sexual assault prior to coming to college may compound the victim's reaction and exacerbate the symptoms they display. Alternately, they may report feeling "numb" as a result of the assault and have no feelings at all. If the student reveals this information to you, a supportive and caring response is required, such as, "It sounds as though this incident on campus has triggered some other memories for you. Dealing with all of these issues at this time may be very difficult. Would you consider talking about it with a professional who works with these types of experiences?"

In addition to campus counseling agencies or outside mental health professionals who specialize in trauma, you may also consider sending the student to a victim center, if one is available. Many campuses have victim advocacy centers that offer specialized counseling and services for victims of sexual assault. Referral to such a center may provide the student with the resources they need. You can say, "I don't know if you are aware, but we have a victim empowerment center on campus. It is near the student health center. From what you told me, I think the staff may be best able to help you determine what your next steps are. Of course, I am still here for you to talk to, and you can come back after seeing what they offer." As stated previously, make this an option for the victim, not an ultimatum. You want the victim to decide if this is an option to pursue. At a time when the victim feels as though all control has been lost, your aim is to return a small amount.

Unintended consequences of sexual assaults include sexually

transmitted infections and pregnancy. The student may need to be referred to a medical center or campus health clinic to be tested for these conditions. Some centers also have rape kits and can collect specimens that may be helpful later in legal proceedings, should the victim decide to go in that direction. Higher education professionals should familiarize themselves with local resources, including centers that have sexual assault nurse examiners or sexual assault response teams. Local professionals who can be of assistance include those working in health care, forensics, the local rape crisis center, law enforcement, and the prosecutor's office. Available health services include "Plan B" pills that can help prevent pregnancy as well as medications to avoid infections, such as chlamydia, herpes simplex virus, and human papillomavirus. However, you should not push victims to participate in this process if they do not want to. Some ways to approach a victim might sound like, "The center downtown has a special unit that helps victims with some of the physical concerns you may have right now, including possible pregnancy and injury or infection. Do you think that is something you want to consider?" or "I was wondering if you would want to take the phone number to the center that helps with medical concerns after someone has been assaulted. I have it here if you want it."

Whether you continue to provide support to the victim on your own or the victim accepts a referral to an agency that specializes in treatment, your interactions with the victim need to be supportive, nonjudgmental, and caring. Sometimes the victim's friends and family may respond in a derisive or negative manner, which can hinder the victim's recovery and contribute to feelings of blame and shame. Make an effort to establish yourself as someone known to assist victims and provide a listening ear, while focusing on connecting them to the professional help they may require for long-term recovery.

Conclusion

Sexual violence and assault are all too common on college and university campuses. Certain activities, including drinking and use of drugs, put victims at risk for sexual assault. Most victims are assaulted by individuals known to them and they are often ashamed to come forward for help. Higher education professionals may be approached by concerned friends of the victim, and thus be in a position to assist victims and refer them for intervention with trauma specialists. These professionals are trained in handling the reactions that result from sexual trauma among students and can provide appropriate treatment and resources. While the United States has begun to address the magnitude of sexual violence and some campuses are engaged in campaigns such as It's On Us, sexual assaults are still occurring at an alarming rate. Survivors need support and services so they can get professional help with their trauma and refocus on their studies and college life. In doing so, they can begin transitioning from a victim to a survivor of sexual assault.

References

Abbey, A., Zawacki, T., Buck, P. O., Clinton, A. M., & McAuslan, P. (2004). Sexual assault and alcohol consumption: What do we know about their relationship and what types of research are still needed? *Aggression and Violent Behavior, 9*(3), 271–303. https://doi.org/10.1016/S1359-1789(03)00011-9

Ahrens, C. E., & Campbell, R. (2000). Assisting rape victims as they recover from rape: The impact on friends. *Journal of Interpersonal Violence, 15*(9), 959–986. https://doi.org/10.1177%2F088626000015009004

Allison, R., & Risman, B. J. (2013). A double standard for "hooking up": How far have we come toward gender equality? *Social Science Research, 42*(5), 1191–1206. https://doi.org/10.1016/j.ssresearch.2013.04.006

American Psychiatric Association. (2013). *Diagnostic and statistical manual of mental disorders* (5th ed.).

Banyard, V. L., Moynihan, M. M., Walsh, W. A., Cohn, E. S., & Ward, S. K. (2010). Friends of survivors: The community impact of unwanted sexual experiences. *Journal of Interpersonal Violence, 25*(2), 242–256. https://doi.org/10.1177/0886260509334407

Bateman, J. L., & Wathen, C. (2015). Understanding rape myths: A guide for counselors working with male survivors of sexual violence. *VISTAS Online*. https://www.counseling.org/docs/default-source/vistas/understanding-rape-myths.pdf?sfvrsn=1cdb432c_8

Black, M. C., Basile, K. C., Breiding, M. J., Smith, S. G., Walters, M. L., Merrick, M. T., Chen, J., & Stevens, M. R. (2011). *The national intimate partner and sexual violence survey: 2010 summary report*. National Center for Injury Prevention and Control, Centers for Disease Control and Prevention. https://www.cdc.gov/violenceprevention/pdf/nisvs_report2010-a.pdf

Bollinger, C., Flintoft, R., Nicoletti, J., Spencer-Thomas, S., & Dvoskina, M. (2018). *Violence goes to college: The authoritative guide to prevention, intervention and response.* Charles C. Thomas.

Boulware, L. E., Cooper, L. A., Ratner, L. E., LaVeist, T. A., & Powe, N. R. (2003). Race and trust in the health care system. *Public Health Reports, 118,* 358–365.

Brewin, C. R. (2007). Autobiographical memory for trauma: Update on four controversies. *Memory, 15*(3), 227–248. https://doi.org/10.1080/09658210701256423

Bryant-Davis, T., Ullman, S. E., Tsong, Y., & Gobin, R. (2011). Surviving the storm: The role of social support and religious coping in sexual assault recovery of African American women. *Violence Against Women, 17*(12), 1601–1618. https://doi.org/10.1177/1077801211436138

Cantor, D., Fisher, B., Chibnall, S., Bruce, C., Townsend, R., Thomas, G., & Lee, H. (2015). *Report on the AAU campus climate survey on sexual assault and sexual misconduct.* Association of American Universities. https://www.aau.edu/sites/default/files/AAU-Files/Key-Issues/Campus-Safety/AAU-Campus-Climate-Survey-FINAL-10-20-17.pdf

Carey, K. B., Durney, S. E., Shepardson, R. L., & Carey, M. P. (2015). Incapacitated and forcible rape of college women: Prevalence across the first year. *Journal of Adolescent Health, 56*(6), 678–680. https://doi.org/10.1016/j.jadohealth.2015.02.018

Coulter, R. W. S., Mair, C., Miller, E., Blosnich, J. R., Matthews, D. D., & McCauley, H. L. (2017). Prevalence of past-year sexual assault victimization among undergraduate students: Exploring differences by and intersections of gender identity, sexual identity, and race/ethnicity. *Prevention Science, 18*(6), 726–736. https://dx.doi.org/10.1007%2Fs11121-017-0762-8

Dick, K. (Director). (2015). *The hunting ground* [Film]. The Weinstein Company.

Engel, B. (2008, September 23). Stop shaming victims of sexual assault for not reporting. *Psychology Today.* https://www.psychologytoday.com/us/blog/the-compassion-chronicles/201809/stop-shaming-victims-sexual-assault-not-reporting

England, P., Allison, P., Li, S., Mark, N., Thompson, J., Budig, M., & Sun, H. (2007). Why are some academic fields tipping toward female? The sex composition of U.S. fields of doctoral degree receipt, 1971–2002. *Sociology of Education, 80*(1), 23–42. https://doi.org/10.1177%2F003804070708000102

Fedina, L., Holmes, J. L., & Backes, B. L. (2016). Campus sexual assault: A systematic review of prevalence research from 2000 to 2015. *Trauma, Violence, & Abuse, 19*(1), 76–93. https://doi.org/10.1177/1524838016631129

Fisher, B. S., Cullen, F. T., & Turner, M. G. (2000). *The sexual victimization of college women* (Publication No. NCJ 182369). U.S. Department of Justice, National Institute of Justice. https://www.ncjrs.gov/App/Publications/abstract.aspx?ID=182369

Fisher, B. S., Daigle, L. E., Cullen, F. T., & Turner, M. G. (2003). Reporting sexual victimization to the police and others: Results from a national-level study of college women. *Criminal Justice and Behavior, 30*(1), 6–38. https://doi.org/10.1177%2F0093854802239161

Ford, J., & Soto-Marquez, J. (2016). Sexual assault victimization among straight, gay/lesbian, and bisexual college students. *Violence and Gender, 3*(2), 107–115. https://doi.org/10.1089/vio.2015.0030

Frankowski, B. L. (2004). Sexual orientation and adolescents. *Pediatrics, 113*(6), 1827–1832. https://doi.org/10.1542/peds.113.6.1827

Gidycz, C. A., Orchowski, L. M., King, C. R., & Rich, C. L. (2008). Sexual victimization and health-risk behaviors: A prospective analysis of college women. *Journal of Interpersonal Violence, 23*(6), 744–763. https://doi.org/10.1177/0886260507313944

Grant, J. M., Mottet, L., Tanis, J. E., Harrison, J., Herman, J., & Keisling, M. (2011). *Injustice at every turn: A report of the national transgender discrimination survey.* National Center for Transgender Equality.

Hardy, A., Young, K., & Holmes, E. (2009). Does trauma memory play a role in the experience of reporting sexual assault during police interviews? An exploratory study. *Memory, 17*(8), 783–788. https://doi.org/10.1080/09658210903081835

Humphrey, J. A., & White, J. W. (2000). Women's vulnerability to sexual assault from adolescence to young adulthood. *Journal of Adolescent Health, 27*(6), 419–424. https://doi.org/10.1016/S1054-139X(00)00168-3

Kirkpatrick, D. G., Koenen, K. C., Ruggiero, K. J., Acierno, R., Galea, S., Resnick, H. S., Roitzsch, J., Boyle, J., & Gelernter, J. (2007). The serotonin transporter genotype and social support and moderation of posttraumatic stress disorder and depression in hurricane-exposed adults. *American Journal of Psychiatry, 164*(11), 1693–1699. https://doi.org/10.1176/appi.ajp.2007.06122007

Krebs, C. P., Lindquist, C. H., Warner, T. D., Fisher, B. S., & Martin, S. L. (2007). *The campus sexual assault (CSA) study: Final report.* National Criminal Justice Reference Service. http://www.ncjrs.gov/pdffiles1/nij/grants/221153.pdf

Krebs, C. P., Lindquist, C. H., Warner, T. D., Fisher, B. S., & Martin, S. L. (2009). The differential risk factors of physically forced and alcohol- or other drug-enabled sexual assault among university women. *Violence and Victims, 24*(3), 302–321. https://doi.org/10.1891/0886-6708.24.3.302

Martin, S. L., Fisher, B. S., Warner, T. D., Krebs, C. P., & Lindquist, C. H. (2011). Women's sexual orientations and their experiences of sexual assault before and during university. *Women's Health Issues, 21*(3), 199–205. https://doi.org/10.1016/j.whi.2010.12.002

Nickerson, A., Steenkamp, M., Aerka, I. M., Salters-Pedneault, K., Carper, T. L., Barnes, J. B., & Litz, B. T. (2013). Prospective investigation of mental health following sexual assault. *Depression and Anxiety, 30*(5), 444–450. https://doi.org/10.1002/da.22023

Orchowski, L. M., Untied, A. S., & Gidycz, C. A. (2013). Factors associated with college women's labeling of sexual victimization. *Violence and Victims, 28*(6), 940–958. https://dx.doi.org/10.1891/0886-6708.VV-D-12-00049

Ottens, A. J., & Hotelling, K. (2001). *Sexual violence on campus: Policies, programs, and perspectives.* Springer.

Paul, L. A., Walsh, K., McCauley, J. L., Ruggiero, K. J., Resnick, H. S., & Kilpatrick, D. G. (2013). College women's experiences with rape disclosure: A national study. *Violence Against Women, 19*(4), 486–502. https://doi.org/10.1177/1077801213487746

Persson, S., Dhingra, K., & Grogan, S. (2018). Attributions of victim blame in stranger and acquaintance rape: A quantitative study. *Journal of Clinical Nursing, 27*(13–14), 2640–2649. https://doi.org/10.1111/jocn.14351

Rape, Abuse, & Incest National Network. (2021). *Victims of sexual violence: Statistics.* https://www.rainn.org/statistics/victims-sexual-violence

Read, J. P., Ouimette, P., White, J., Colder, C., & Farrow, S. (2011). Rates of *DSM–IV–TR* trauma exposure and posttraumatic stress disorder among newly matriculated college students. *Psychological Trauma: Theory, Research, Practice, and Policy, 3*(2), 148–156. https://doi.org/10.1037/a0021260

Reed, E., Amaro, H., Matsumoto, A., & Kaysen, D. (2009). The relation between interpersonal violence and substance use among a sample of university students: Examination of the role of victim and perpetrator substance use. *Addictive Behaviors, 34*(3), 316–318. https://doi.org/10.1016/j.addbeh.2008.10.015

Rennison, C. M., & Dodge, M. (2012). Police impersonation: Pretenses and predators. *American Journal of Criminal Justice, 37*(4), 505–522. https://doi.org/10.1007/s12103-011-9153-z

Roodman, A. A., & Clum, G. A. (2001). Revictimization rates and method variance: A meta-analysis. *Clinical Psychology Review, 21*(2), 183–204. https://doi.org/10.1016/S0272-7358(99)00045-8

Sabina, C., & Ho, L. Y. (2014). Campus and college victim responses to sexual assault and dating violence: Disclosure, service utilization, and service provision. *Trauma, Violence, & Abuse, 15*(3), 201–226. https://doi.org/10.1177/1524838014521322

Sinozich, S., & Langton, L. (2014). *Rape and sexual assault victimization among college-age females, 1995–2013.* U.S. Department of Justice. https://bjs.ojp.gov/content/pub/pdf/rsavcaf9513.pdf

Turchik, J. A., Probst, D. R., Irvin, C. R., Chau, M., & Gidycz, C. A. (2010). Prediction of sexual assault experiences in college women based on rape scripts: A prospective analysis. *Psychology of Violence, 1*, 76–83. https://doi.org/10.1037/2152-0828.1.S.76

Ullman, S. E., & Filipas, H. H. (2001). Correlates of formal and informal support seeking in sexual assaults victims. *Journal of Interpersonal Violence, 16*(10), 1028–1047. https://doi.org/10.1177/088626001016010004

Ullman, S. E., Filipas, H. H., Townsend, S. M., & Starzynski, L. L. (2007). Psychosocial correlates of PTSD symptom severity in sexual assault survivors. *Journal of Traumatic Stress, 20*(5), 821–831. https://doi.org/10.1002/jts.20290

Untied, A. S., Orchowski, L. M., Mastroleo, N., & Gidycz, C. A. (2012). College students' social reactions to the victim in a hypothetical sexual assault scenario: The role of victim and perpetrator alcohol use. *Violence and Victims, 27*(6), 957–972. https://doi.org/10.1891/0886-6708.27.6.957

Weare, S. (2018). 'Oh you're a guy, how could you be raped by a woman, that makes no sense': Towards a case for legally recognising and labelling 'forced-to-penetrate' cases as rape. *International Journal of Law in Context, 14*(1), 110–131. https://doi.org/10.1017/S1744552317000179

Wilcox, H. C., Storr, C. L., & Breslau, N. (2009). Posttraumatic stress disorder and suicide attempts in a community sample of urban American young adults. *Archives of General Psychiatry, 66*(3), 305–311. https://doi.org/10.1001/archgenpsychiatry.2008.557

Zinzow, H. M., Amstadter, A. B., McCauley, J. L., Ruggiero, K. J., Resnick, H. S., & Kilpatrick, D. G. (2011). Self-rated health in relation to rape and mental health disorders in a national sample of college women. *Journal of American College Health, 59*(7), 588–594. https://doi.org/10.1080/07448481.2010.520175

CHAPTER 11

Interpersonal Violence

This chapter will discuss the different types of abuse and interpersonal violence that can occur in relationships. Students may be the victims of stalking, violence, or emotional abuse. Interpersonal violence can occur in same-sex or heterosexual relationships and may even take place after the relationship has ended. The chapter will present the signs and symptoms someone in an abusive relationship might display. Higher education professionals should acquire a certain level of expertise on and comfort with recognizing these signs, as students themselves may not realize that they are in an unhealthy relationship. Interpersonal violence is a sensitive and often difficult subject to talk about. The chapter will advise higher education professionals on approaching this complex topic and address how to support students in unhealthy relationships.

Basic Signs and Symptoms of Interpersonal Violence

> **Case Study**
>
> Katherine had begun dating Benjamin in high school. She was a much better student than he was, so it came as no surprise when she got admitted to the most competitive state university. Benjamin, however, stayed home and attended community college. At first, during her adjustment to college, roommates, and campus life, it was nice having Benjamin to talk to after a long day of classes. Over time, Katherine began to make friends and go out at night. She always told Benjamin where she was going and what she was doing. Soon, he began to get angry when she did not answer his calls or return his texts immediately. Though she tried to reassure him that she was often studying in the library or out with her girlfriends, he got angry and accused her of being unfaithful. Their phone calls often ended in fights, and he would call her a whore or a slut. Katherine began to turn down offers from her friends to go out and stayed in her room most nights. She started to feel a bit depressed and hopeless about the situation with Benjamin.

Interpersonal violence (IPV), historically referred to as *domestic violence*, is when one partner uses power and control over another through physical, sexual, or emotional abuse; economic control; isolation; or other coercive means (see Chapter 10 for more on sexual victimization). Traditionally thought to include only physical abuse (pushing, shoving, hitting, or beating) in marriages, IPV has expanded in definition to include two people who are or were in a relationship. Although the overt physically aggressive acts are more obvious in violence, those who perpetrate IPV may also verbally threaten, demean, or control their partners. Controlling behaviors can include intimidation in the form of threats of physical violence or destruction of property (e.g., breaking something important to the victim). Other, more subtle forms of control include insisting someone change their preferences, interests, hobbies, career choices, or lifestyle. Naturally, people may change over time, but insistence from a partner that someone stop doing something they really enjoy is a form of control.

Some perpetrators of IPV use isolation to control what the victim does. Examples include limiting the partner's involvement in the outside world and controlling where or with whom the partner goes. IPV can also include forms of emotional abuse such as name calling and humiliation. In the case above, Benjamin engaged in many of these behaviors. People in healthy relationships respect and trust one another. They share decision-making power. In unhealthy relationships, power is unbalanced, and one partner tries to control the other. Table 11.1 presents the differences between healthy and unhealthy relationships.

In recent years, the epidemic of campus sexual assault, stalking, and IPV has gained national attention. The Association of American Universities (Cantor et al., 2019) found that 8% of college students reported IPV. Forty-three percent of college women reported experiencing abusive behaviors from their partner (Knowledge Networks, 2011). The American College Health Association (ACHA, 2022) survey of college students found that 9% of respondents reported that their partners talked down to them, insulted them, and made them feel bad; 5% reported their partners restricted their contact with other people; and 3% reported their partners pushed, grabbed, shoved, kicked, hit, bit, or choked them without their consent. In addition to physical harm, IPV puts students at risk of having mental health problems and contributes to poor academic performance.

Table 11.1
Healthy versus Unhealthy Relationships

Healthy relationships	Unhealthy relationships
Equality – Partners share decisions and responsibilities. They discuss roles to make sure they are fair and equal.	**Control** – One partner makes all the decisions and tells the other what to do or tells the other person what to wear or who to spend time with.
Honesty – Partners share their dreams, fears, and concerns with each other. They tell each other how they feel and share important information.	**Dishonesty** – One partner lies to or keeps information from the other. One partner steals from the other.
Physical safety – Partners feel physically safe in the relationship and respect each other's space.	**Physical abuse** – One partner uses force to get their way (for example, hitting, slapping, grabbing, shoving).
Respect – Partners treat each other like they want to be treated and accept each other's opinions, friends, and interests. They listen to each other.	**Disrespect** – One partner makes fun of opinions and interests of the other partner. He or she may destroy something that belongs to the other partner.
Comfort – Partners feel safe with each other and respect each other's differences. They realize when they're wrong and are not afraid to apologize. Partners can "be themselves" with each other.	**Intimidation** – One partner tries to control every aspect of the other's life. One partner may attempt to keep his or her partner from friends and family or threaten violence or a breakup.
Sexual respectfulness – Partners never force sexual activity or insist on doing something the other isn't comfortable with.	**Sexual abuse** – One partner pressures or forces the other into sexual activity against their will or without their consent.
Independence – Neither partner depends on the other for an identity. Partners maintain friendships outside of the relationship. Either partner has the right to end the relationship.	**Dependence** – One partner feels that they can't live without the other. They may threaten to do something drastic if the relationship ends.
Humor – The relationship is enjoyable for both partners. Partners laugh and have fun.	**Hostility** – One partner may "walk on eggshells" to avoid upsetting the other. Teasing is mean-spirited.

Note. From *Choose Respect Community Action Kit* (p. 7), by Centers for Disease Control and Prevention, 2006. In the public domain.

Dating violence is a particular threat to college students because many enter into their first serious romantic relationship during these years and may lack fully developed communication and relationship skills (Kaukinen, 2014). These factors, along with the autonomy that college life provides and sexual intimacy, likely influence the continuum of violence within and across intimate relationships (Kaukinen, 2014).

Young adults do not have a lot of relationship experience, and it's likely that if they had unhealthy relationships in high school, they'll continue to experience them in college. Mason and Smithey (2012) found that the amount of time a couple has been dating increases the likelihood of IPV in college couples. The longer the relationship, the more time partners have to gain knowledge about the other and become familiar with one another within the relationship. This closeness allows the perpetrator to be in position to do emotional harm via psychological aggression and, potentially, physical harm through minor assault. Kaukinen (2014) concluded that expectations of monogamy, levels of sexual and physical intimacy, and the intensity of commitment are all factors that shape the meaning of intimate relationships. These factors are likely to affect the level of sexual jealousy and the need for power and control by both men and women, which may be expressed through violence in the relationship.

Case Study

Jane met Rachel at college, and it was not long before they began dating. While Jane was comfortable with her sexuality, she had not formally come out to her parents, who were very religious and conservative. Jane and Rachel had a lot in common and enjoyed going to parties, attending concerts, and hanging out with other students. Over time, Rachel began to become verbally abusive to Jane. It started with small comments about Jane's weight or something she was wearing. One evening, Rachel got incredibly angry when Jane was late meeting her for dinner. Rachel began to yell at Jane and accused her of being unfaithful. One night when Jane had to stay late at her chemistry lab to finish a project, Rachel slapped her when she returned home and called her a whore. Jane approached the topic of breaking up, but Rachel threatened to "out" Jane to her parents.

The idea that only college women are victims of IPV, at the hands of male partners, is a fallacy. Kaukinen et al. (2012) found that college dating violence involves both men and women as victims and perpetrators and that the aggression often occurs within the context of a mutually violent relationship. IPV is also present in same-sex relationships. In a study by Edwards and Sylaska (2013), 20% of the students who were involved in a same-sex relationship reported physical IPV victimization within their current relationship. In a sample of more than 300 college students, Edwards et al. (2015) found that sexual-minority students reported the following rates of IPV perpetration: physical violence (19.9%), psychological abuse (12.5%), and sexual violence (10.5%). Snyder et al. (2018) found that, on average, students who identified as LGBTQIA+ (male and female) were significantly more likely to experience IPV than their heterosexual counterparts. As seen in the case of Jane, in same sex relationships, "outing" or threatening to reveal one partner's sexual orientation may be used as a tool of abuse in IPV and may also serve to decrease the likelihood of help-seeking by the victim.

Many theories about interpersonal violence abound, though one belief is that those who as children may have witnessed violence among their parents are more likely to be involved in a violent relationship as adults. In a meta-analysis, Smith-Marek et al. (2015) found that men who had experienced family-of-origin violence were more likely to become perpetrators of IPV, while women who experienced family-of-origin violence were more likely to be victims. Witnessing this type of relationship may make it seem like an "acceptable" form of conflict resolution. Men may learn negative attitudes toward women in their families and have been reinforced socially for sexual promiscuity. Peer support of violence, patriarchal attitudes, personal beliefs, alcohol use and abuse, hostility, childhood abuse, and low self-esteem are all factors related to IPV (Lawson, 2013; Mason & Smithey, 2012).

Stalking

IPV also includes threats or stalking. Stalking consists of a series of actions that make the victim feel afraid or in danger. Some common examples of stalking behaviors include showing up uninvited; following the victim; sending unwanted gifts or messages; monitoring the victim's email and computer use; or threatening to hurt the victim or the victim's family and friends (Bruns, 2020). Social media contact, texts, and email can be used to threaten a victim. Other behaviors include spying on a partner, checking social media to see what a partner is doing, and calling a partner who has requested not to be called. Another form of stalking is cyberstalking, which takes place via electronic communications, such as text messages or emails that are harassing and frightening. Cyberstalking can also include collecting information about someone (e.g., incriminating photos) to use against them. The highest rates of stalking are among 18- to 24-year-olds (Breiding et al., 2014), so it is no surprise that it happens on college campuses. Because stalking can escalate over time, it should always be taken very seriously.

ACHA (2022) found that 4% of students reported being a victim of stalking, but other studies have found rates as high as 38% (Shorey et al., 2015). Many victims are stalked by a current or former partner (Krebs et al., 2007). In their study, White and Carmody (2018) found that college women were more likely than men to report cyberstalking, but no respondents reported the problem to the police. Common examples in the ACHA (2022) study included the stalker waiting outside the victim's classroom, residence, or office, or repeated emails/phone calls. Stalkers can also live in the same residence hall, making avoiding them difficult. Lambert et al. (2013) stated that perceptions of stalking are important, as some stalkers may not realize that they are stalking and instead view their behavior as simply pursuing a relationship. Cass and Rosay (2012) reported that some college students do not view stalking by ex-intimates as predatory but rather an expression of love and adoration ("He loves me so much, he can't let go. That is why he waits outside for me."). It is possible that some victims, although they feel threatened, may not view the stalking as illegal, and this perception may affect whether incidents are reported to police. Additionally, it has been found that law enforcement may not take stalking by an ex-intimate partner as seriously as they would stalking by a stranger (McKeon, et al., 2015). Being stalked can be an exhausting, terrifying, and troubling experience.

Students can be considered victims if they experienced at least one of the stalking behaviors mentioned on at least two separate occasions. In addition, the student must have feared for their safety or that of a family member as a result of the stalker's behavior or have experienced additional threatening behaviors that would cause a reasonable person to feel fear. Although some research has shown women as more likely to be victims after termination of a relationship, Shorey et al. (2015) suggested that both men and women are equally likely to be victims during intact relationships.

Approaching the Issue With Students

Higher education professionals must be equipped to screen for victimization and recognize that the experience and impact of IPV can affect students in a variety of ways. IPV can involve substance abuse, mental health issues, and sexual risk-taking, and it can have a negative impact on students' academic success and engagement (Kaukinen, 2014). It may be baffling to you, as a higher education professional, why a student would stay in an abusive relationship, but your role is not to judge the student or give advice. This may be harder than it sounds, as it is often difficult to remain calm and quiet when you hear about abuse of any kind. It is critical to keep an open mind and listen if the student begins to open up.

Forming a solid, trusting relationship with the victim will be the first and most important step. Due to the trauma perpetrated by someone they know and love, victims are likely to have trust issues. Most victims will not come forward and report the abusive nature of the relationship. College students are away from home, lacking social support, and the abuse may leave them feeling confused and alone. Student victims often fear that they will get in trouble for the abuse. Ameral et al. (2020) found many barriers to help-seeking among victims, including the belief that it is a personal matter and one not serious enough to discuss. Some victims also did not seek help, as they too had engaged in violence toward their partner at one point and fear they will be judged. There are also situations where the student may lose a scholarship if the abuse is reported. Take, for example, a student who is dating a college athlete on scholarship. If the athlete were to be reported for IPV, this behavior might violate the code of conduct required to maintain the scholarship, resulting in dismissal from the university. So, the higher education professional will have to be alert to statements made about the relationship to determine if it may be abusive.

Female college students have been found to seek help for IPV more often than male college students (Ameral et al., 2020). This may be due to cultural norms that typically portray women as victims more often than men. Men may have difficulty thinking of themselves as victims and thus not seek help. Female victims who are still dating the perpetrator were less likely to seek help, but if they experienced multiple incidents of stalking, they were likely to seek help. Male victims of stalking have great difficulty in reporting and acknowledging their victimization

As with other conditions covered in this book, the higher education professional must believe the victim and listen empathically.

Even trained health professionals will have difficulty addressing the issue of IPV. They may feel uncomfortable, worry that they may offend the victim, and fear the issue is outside their scope of work. It is important to keep in mind that inquiring about the student's safety may be a relief for the victim who has been suffering in silence and is unsure of how to bring it up.

Students with few peer supports are likely to remain in unhealthy relationships. Thus, the higher education professional may be the confidante and listening ear the student needs. Remaining nonjudgmental is a key factor in getting a student to disclose the matter. It is easy to think, "Why would she put up with him?" as a student talks about an abusive boyfriend. However, these situations and the personal dynamics are often complicated. This complexity is also why victims require more intensive counseling than a higher education professional can provide. The professional must not jump in to give advice or tell their own story (e.g., "You need to leave her and find someone who will really love you" or "I, too, had a partner who used to put me down"). The focus must remain on helping the student understand that no one deserves to be abused and it's not their fault. One approach is, "I am worried about how you feel in this relationship. Here are resources when you're ready. I encourage you to make a call. But I want you to know that this is your situation, and you know what is best for you. Is there anything I can do to help?" Share information with students about relevant services and how they can be of help.

Supporting a student who is in an IPV relationship or who is a victim of stalking is likely not a one-time event. You may have to help over a long period of time as the student slowly moves toward making a decision or ending the relationship. Though it may seem easy to tell someone to leave an abusive relationship, only the victim can make that choice and decide when they're ready. You may want to say, "It's hard to know what to do. You are thinking a lot about the good times you have. But you are also scared when Sam behaves like they did the other night. It is your decision, and I am here for you no matter what you decide." It is critical not to get angry with the student who chooses to stay in the relationship. Higher education professionals should want to remain open to the student returning in the future to talk about the relationship. If the student feels that the professional will be accepting only if the relationship ends (conditional acceptance), then they may avoid returning for help or guidance. Remember: Don't push victims into doing anything. Not only is such behavior controlling and disempowering, but victims are less likely to follow through.

LGBTQIA+ victims of IPV may face additional challenges. They are more vulnerable to IPV due to a perceived lower likelihood to report (Snyder et al., 2018). They may not be "out" to their families and thus fear disclosing the violence. Fear of not being taken seriously or believed, or concern over encountering anti-gay attitudes may also impact their willingness to talk about the IPV. Many colleges now provide "safe spaces" or "safe zone" programs for the LGBTQIA+ student community. These areas are often marked with rainbows or other inclusive images. All higher education professionals should be allies for LGBTQIA+ students and provide a safe haven for these students to talk. One way to approach a suspected victim of IPV who is LGBTQIA+ is to say, "I am worried about some of the things you say about your relationship. Are you fearful of talking about it and letting others know you are in a gay relationship?"

When you suspect a student is being stalked, a necessary first step is educating them about stalking. As mentioned earlier, many students may not realize what exactly constitutes stalking behavior. Typically, experts recommend that the victim not confront the stalker but instead keep a record of the stalker's actions: the day and time of each incident and what happened at each event (e.g., left flowers at my room, called me 10 times in a row, showed up at my class). Ultimately, if the student feels threatened, the student should contact the police.

In some instances, the victim may want to obtain a restraining order to ensure that the perpetrator will stay away. The higher education professional can provide these resources to the student: "Aisha, I am worried about Leon's behavior lately and how he keeps showing up at your classes. Here is the campus police number you should call if you feel unsafe. Can you please put it in your phone now?"

If a student describes a stalking situation, it is best to explore their reaction and then refer to a center on campus that may assist. Many campuses have victim empowerment centers or similar places devoted to helping students who have been victims of IPV or sexual violence (see Chapter 10). In cases of IPV or stalking, it is important to listen to victims, show support, and never blame them. Avoid the use of "why" questions (e.g., "Why do you stay with her?" or "Why do you let him treat you like that?"). See Table 11.2 for guidance on how to talk to a victim.

Table 11.2

Things Not to Say to Victims of IPV

Do not blame the victim. It is the perpetrator's behavior that is wrong.
Do not make promises you can't keep ("I'll make sure he never hurts you again").
Do not pressure the victim to leave the relationship. Review choices with the victim.
Do not underestimate the danger that the victim could be in.
Do not put down the perpetrator. Focus on the behavior, not personality. Remember, the victim has complicated feelings for the perpetrator.
Do not give up on the victim. Be patient and be there for when the victim is ready and able to open up and make some changes.

If you suspect that a student may be the victim of IPV or stalking, you will want to assess their safety immediately. You may want to ask about the student's living situation and social support networks. Has the student shared with friends concerns about the relationship? Are the partners living together? How violent has the perpetrator become? Ensure that students have a hotline number to call before they leave your office. You may also want to discuss with the victim a safety plan, which is what specific steps they'd follow if they felt threatened or afraid—for example, determining where to go for the night if the ex-partner keeps showing up at their residence hall or work, or ways the student can alter daily routines to avoid the stalker for a day or two. Is there a friend or relative they can bring with them when they go out, so they are not alone? Unfortunately, in stalking cases, the victims—not the stalkers—may be forced to make changes in their behavior. It will be important for the victim to tell others about the stalking—for example, telling the security desk at the residence hall not to let the stalker into the building. Informing friends and other confidantes about the situation, so they can provide support, help, and be on the lookout for the stalker, is critical to ensuring safety.

When and How to Make a Referral to Counseling

Once a higher education professional confirms (or strongly suspects) that a student is the victim of IPV, a referral should be made to a trained professional. Given the potential risk of continued violence (and in extreme cases, fatality), all cases of IPV must be taken seriously. Letting the student know that there are services for this type of work can be a starting point: "Jan, you have told me a lot about what happens with Rod. I am concerned about you and wonder if you might be willing to talk to a professional, someone who is trained in these issues." Remind the student that the services are confidential and that the student can decide which services to use or how much information to share. In other words, students will be presented with options about their situation and relationship and can make a choice. No professional should tell or insist the student take a certain action. Emphasize the potential harm that may come to the victim and how you want to be sure they are safe:

> *John, it seems Emily is getting more and more aggressive and physical with you. I am really worried about your safety. I want to help you, but there are others on campus who have much more training and expertise in this area. Would you be willing to get some different help with this issue?*
>
> *Sarah, I see how upset you are most days about the relationship with Jordan. You seem tearful and are having a hard time in classes. I think this is a bigger issue than I may be able to help you with. Would you be willing to call the campus counseling center? I can help you with that if you want.*

In cases of stalking, the higher education professional must educate the student that this behavior constitutes a crime and then point the student toward options. You may want to say, "You seem really scared by Toni's behavior, and I am too. I think it would be good for you to talk to someone at a center we have on campus. I am worried that Toni may do something to hurt you. It's important for you to find out about the options you have." The U.S. federal government, all 50 states, and the District of Columbia have enacted criminal laws to address stalking, and counselors or victims' advocates trained in this type of work are in the best position to help victims.

Conclusion

College life can be the start of intimate relationships for many students. Out from under parental authority and immersed in a world of same-age peers, relationships are quick to form. For some students, these relationships may be unhealthy and involve control and physical violence. Often, students cannot recognize the early signs of an unhealthy relationship and may misinterpret their partner's actions. Stalking is one form of interpersonal violence that students may experience and can be very frightening. The shame experienced by victims who are in abusive relationships may contribute to maintaining their silence so that others do not become aware of what is happening. Higher education professionals should be alert to signs of interpersonal violence and be proactive in prevention efforts on campus. Knowing all the available resources and legal options for students who are involved in relationships where violence takes place will assist with making successful referrals. It is important to get students help and ensure their safety on campus.

References

Ameral, V., Palm Reed, K. M., & Hines, D. A. (2020). An analysis of help-seeking patterns among college student victims of sexual assault, dating violence, and stalking. *Journal of Interpersonal Violence, 35*(23–24), 5311–5335. https://doi.org/10.1177/0886260517721169

American College Health Association. (2022). *American College Health Association–National college health assessment III: Reference group data report fall 2021.* https://www.acha.org/documents/ncha/NCHA-III_FALL_2021_REFERENCE_GROUP_DATA_REPORT.pdf

Breiding, M. J., Smith, S. G., Basile, K. C., Walters, M. L., Chen, J., & Merrick, M. T. (2014). Prevalence and characteristics of sexual violence, stalking, and intimate partner violence victimization—National intimate partner and sexual violence survey, United States, 2011. *MMWR. Surveillance Summaries, 63*(8), 1–18.

Bruns, K. (2020). Sexual victimization. In D. Paladino, L. Gonzalez, & J. Watson (Eds.), *College counseling and student development: Theory, practice, and campus collaboration* (pp. 431–442). American Counseling Association.

Cantor, C., Fisher, B., Chibnall, S., Harps, S., Townsend, R., Thomas, G., Lee, H., Kranz, V., Herbison, R., & Madden, K. (2019). *Report on the AAU campus climate survey on sexual assault and sexual misconduct.* Westat. https://ira.virginia.edu/sites/ias.virginia.edu/files/aau-uva-campus-climate-survey-report-2019.pdf

Cass, A. I., & Rosay, A. B. (2012). College student perceptions of criminal justice system responses to stalking. *Sex Roles: A Journal of Research, 66*(5–6), 392–404. https://doi.org/10.1007/s11199-011-9934-3

Edwards, K. M., & Sylaska, K. M. (2013). The perpetration of intimate partner violence among LGBTQ college youth: The role of minority stress. *Journal of Youth and Adolescence, 42*, 1721–1731. https://doi.org/10.1007/s10964-012-9880-6

Edwards, K. M., Sylaska, K. M., Barry, J. E., Moynihan, M. M., Banyard, V. L., Cohn, E. S., Walsh, W. A., & Ward, S. K. (2015). Physical dating violence, sexual violence, and unwanted pursuit victimization: A comparison of incidence rates among sexual-minority and heterosexual college students. *Journal of Interpersonal Violence, 30*(4), 580–600. https://doi.org/10.1177/0886260514535260

Kaukinen, C. (2014). Dating violence among college students: The risk and protective factors. *Trauma, Violence, & Abuse, 15*(4), 283–296. https://doi.org/10.1177/1524838014521321

Kaukinen, C., Gover, A. R., & Hartman, J. L. (2012). College women's experiences of dating violence in casual and exclusive relationships. *American Journal of Criminal Justice, 37*, 146–162. https://doi.org/10.1007/s12103-011-9113-7

Knowledge Networks. (2011). *2011 college dating violence and abuse poll*. Fifth and Pacific Companies. http://www.loveisrespect.org/pdf/College_Dating_And_Abuse_Final_Study.pdf

Krebs, C. P., Lindquist, C. H., Warner, T. D., Fisher, B. S., & Martin, S. L. (2007). *The campus sexual assault study*. National Institute of Justice. https://www.ncjrs.gov/pdffiles1/nij/grants/221153.pdf

Lambert, E. G., Smith, B., Geistman, J., Cluse-Tolar, T., & Jiang, S. (2013). Do men and women differ in their perceptions of stalking: An exploratory study among college students. *Violence and Victims, 28*(2), 195–209. https://doi.org/10.1891/0886-6708.09-201

Lawson, D. (2013). *Family violence: Explanations and evidence-based clinical practice*. American Counseling Association.

Mason, B., & Smithey, M. (2012). The effects of academic and interpersonal stress on dating violence among college students: A test of classical strain theory. *Journal of Interpersonal Violence, 27*(5), 974–986. http://doi.org/10.1177/0886260511423257

McKeon, B., McEwan, T. E., & Luebbers, S. (2015). "It's not really stalking if you know the person": Measuring community attitudes that normalize, justify and minimize stalking. *Psychiatry, Psychology and Law, 22*(2), 291–306. https://doi.org/10.1080/13218719.2014.945637

Shorey, R. C., Cornelius, T. L., & Strauss, C. (2015). Stalking in college student dating relationships: A descriptive investigation. *Journal of Family Violence, 30*, 935–942. http://doi.org/10.1007/s10896-015-9717-7

Smith-Marek, E. N., Cafferky, B., Dharnidharka, P., Mallory, A. B., Dominguez, M., High, J., Stith, S. M., & Mendez, M. (2015). Effects of childhood experiences of family violence on adult partner violence: A meta-analytic review. *Journal of Family Theory & Review, 7*(4), 498–519. https://doi.org/10.1111/jftr.12113

Snyder, J., Scherer, H., & Fisher, B. (2018). Interpersonal violence among college students: Does sexual orientation impact risk of victimization? *Journal of School Violence, 17*(1),1–15, https://doi.org/10.1080/15388220.2016.1190934

White, W. E., & Carmody, D. (2018). Preventing online victimization: College students' views on intervention and prevention. *Journal of Interpersonal Violence, 33*(14), 2291–2307. https://doi.org/10.1177/0886260515625501

CHAPTER 12

Substance Abuse

This chapter includes current, relevant literature on the use of substances among student populations. This chapter aims to help the reader gain an understanding of commonly used substances, including depressants, stimulants, cannabis, and hallucinogens. Readers will be challenged to explore their attitudes toward substance use and gain skills in identifying abuse among students. Readers will develop the ability to distinguish between recreational use and substance abuse that can interfere with functioning. Given the level of denial among substance users, professionals will be guided in approaches they can use to gain information about the impact of substance use on students' well-being. The chapter explores how to make an appropriate referral and the types of treatment available.

Basic Signs and Symptoms of Substance Disorders

While college is intended to be a time of intense study and focus on learning, it has also become a place of excessive substance use for many students. The abuse of substances by college students is one of the primary concerns among those who work at college counseling centers (Reetz et al., 2016). A survey administered by the American College Health Association (ACHA, 2022) found that 6% of college students reported using alcohol, 36% used marijuana, and 7% used prescription drugs that were not prescribed to them. Factors associated with college life that appear to contribute to the heavy substance use include unstructured time, lack of parental control, accessibility of alcohol, and inconsistent and at times lax policing of the problem (National Institute on Alcohol Abuse and Alcoholism, 2020). The culture of college parties, replete with alcohol and drugs, has been portrayed in social media and Hollywood movies, and often the unfortunate consequences for some students are reported in the news.

Despite this picture of rampant substance use, consumption of alcohol and drugs does vary. For example, 24% of students in the ACHA (2022) study reported complete abstinence from alcohol and 59% reported never using marijuana. Some students may abstain due to their own recovery (less than 2% in the ACHA survey), family addiction patterns, or religious beliefs (Likis-Werle, 2020). Many colleges have residence halls or floors devoted to substance-free living (see the sidebox "Substance Free and Healthy Living at College" for a description of one college program). Without parental guidance and with few interactions with adults, some college youth may experiment with substances, which can be considered normative. This chapter will focus on those students whose use may become excessive.

> **Substance Free and Healthy Living at College**
>
> Lehigh University has the CHOICE community, which is committed to a substance-free and healthy lifestyle where students come together to engage in responsible and healthy decision making. The CHOICE community focuses on a mentorship approach in which students, in collaboration with Lehigh After Dark, can explore their Lehigh experience without the pressure of experimenting with substance use. CHOICE community members choose not to use alcohol or tobacco products or to engage in other activities that fall out of a community definition of "healthy living." This community is one of mutual respect and understanding, and while it is not a strictly noise-free environment, those who visit this community are asked to respect community guidelines and CHOICE standards.

The National Institute on Drug Abuse (2020) explained why people take drugs or become addicted. First, using drugs makes one feel good. There is no denying the range of physical effects that are caused by substances: euphoria, happiness, increased self-confidence, relaxation, or increased energy. Drugs also help one deal with the stress of college life. Using substances from time to time can help one relax and not worry for a while. Finally, some drug use is related to curiosity. This may be particularly applicable to college students who are succumbing to peer pressure and are also at a stage of life where they are still exploring who they are.

Research shows, however, that college campuses are not parties all the time for everyone. College students' substance use tends to occur in a routine pattern that consists mostly of weekend use, with elevated consumption at the start of semesters when the workload is relatively light and then reduced consumption during exams (Tremblay et al., 2010). Some college populations are at higher risk than others for use of substances, such as those who are part of Greek life, athletes, LGBTQIA+ individuals, and students who have mental health issues (Likis-Werle, 2020). "High risk" means the person tends to use substances more frequently than others in their peer group and in large amounts and continues to use despite experiencing negative consequences.

> **Case Study**
>
> Hannah was on the swim team and had an athletic scholarship. While she studied as much as she could, she never had enough time to do all the reading required of her. Her grades were starting to drop, and she was worried about being put on academic probation. She looked particularly stressed out one day at practice. Her teammate, Adina, approached her and asked what was wrong. Hannah complained that she did not have enough hours in the day to work out, practice, and study. Adina shared with her the secret for staying up late and studying—"the study drug." Adina told her that lots of people on the team use it to help them study, and she added that it helps you lose weight, an added bonus for swimming. The "study drug" Adina was referring to was Adderall, a prescription stimulant used with individuals who have attention deficit disorder and need help focusing (Essig Aberg et al., n.d.). Hannah was happy to find a solution to her study problem. Before long, Hannah found herself dependent on the drug and often unable to sleep at night.

College athletes face unique demands at school. They have to balance schoolwork, practice, training, and competition. The challenges of being a student-athlete puts them at elevated risk for problematic substance use with both alcohol and other recreational drugs, but also with performance-enhancing substances, which are a concern at all levels of athletics (Buckman et al., 2013). Buckman et al. (2013) found that male college athletes who used performance-enhancing drugs were also more likely to use alcohol (in large quantities and bingeing), marijuana, cigarettes, and cocaine. Druckman et al. (2015) found serious underreporting of substance use by college athletes and concluded that this indicates substantial social desirability and/or fear of disclosure. Many students may be on athletic scholarships and fear disclosure. In Hannah's case, she was concerned about losing her scholarship if her grades dropped, so she turned to the "study drug." Given the National Collegiate Athletic Association's (NCAA, 2021) policy on substance use among college athletes, it is not surprising that athletes underreport use. This has implications for the higher education professional who encounters these students, since student-athletes may gravely underreport their substance use.

Compared to their nonathlete counterparts, college student-athletes are more at risk for unhealthy drinking patterns and negative consequences (e.g., driving under the influence, academic and relationship problems; Donohue et al., 2016). A 2018 NCAA study on the drinking habits of student-athletes found that 77% reported drinking alcohol in the last year. Almost half (42%) of student-athletes reported binge drinking, which is defined as 4 or more drinks for women and 5 or more drinks for men. The highest rates of binge drinking by sport were among lacrosse, hockey, and swimming (for both male and female athletes). While some research shows student-athletes intensifying their drinking over time, freshman student-athletes are at particular risk of fatality or serious injury due to alcohol intoxication (Borsari et al., 2007).

It appears that, for some students, being part of a fraternity involves excessive drinking. McCabe et al. (2018) found that male fraternity members who lived in fraternity houses during college had the highest levels of binge drinking and marijuana use relative to their peers who were not members. (According to McCabe et al., these patterns of drinking continue beyond college, with 45% meeting the criteria for alcohol use disorders at age 35.) The phenomenon results from both selection and socialization effects, where those who are heavy drinkers before college may choose to join a fraternity or sorority known for heavy drinking, and being part of Greek life serves to increase their heavy drinking (McCabe et al., 2018). Drinking to intoxication by college students was found to be most prevalent in Greek-life settings (63%) when compared to other settings both on and off campus, and fraternity and sorority houses were most likely to have a keg (Marzell et al., 2015).

Reed et al. (2010) found that compared to heterosexual students, LGBTQIA+ students were more likely to report recent illicit drug use and negative consequences from their alcohol or drug use. These authors also suggested that violence, safety, and stress experienced by these students partially contribute to their substance use. These findings with regard to social stress (both on and off campus) were confirmed by Manning et al. (2012) with LGBTQIA+ students at community colleges. However, the findings suggest that LGBTQIA+ students may also be using alcohol and other drugs for similar reasons as heterosexual students, including identity-related or emotional, financial, or social-environmental issues. Research has shown that bisexual men and women had a greater likelihood of alcohol and other drug use than heterosexual and gay/lesbian students, and bisexual women had the highest levels of use among all of the sexual orientation groups (Kerr et al., 2014). Higher education professionals will want to be aware of the unique stressors that many college students experience as well as their socialization processes on campus.

Alcohol

Drinking has become synonymous with many college students' experiences, although almost 50% of college students are under the legal drinking age (Substance Abuse and Mental Health Services Administration [SAMHSA], 2021). Alcohol is considered a central nervous system (CNS) depressant. The behavioral result is often slurred speech, disinhibition, disorientation, and other "drunken" behaviors. While the initial effects can feel quite good, overdose or too much alcohol affects the areas of the CNS that control breathing, heart rate, and blood pressure (Lewis, 2015).

Case Study

Peter loved going to a college that boasted a nationally winning football team. During the fall season, most Saturdays were spent getting ready for the game. "Kegs and Eggs" is what the students affectionately called these mornings. Although the game did not start until the afternoon, by 8 a.m. Peter was with his friends making breakfast, but mostly drinking beer. Someone would get a keg and the drinking and drinking games began. Often by noon, he was drunk and had a hard time standing up. Most of his friends were intoxicated too. They would sometimes be too drunk to make it to the stadium for the game. He would sleep it off most of Sunday but be back in class by Monday.

Grossbard et al. (2016) stated, "Heavy drinking and alcohol-related consequences continue to be significant public health problems for college students across the United States" (p. 75). According to the SAMHSA (2019) national survey on drug use and health, 38% of college students reported heavy episodic or binge drinking in the past month. Peter is a good example of a college student who binge drinks. While he may not drink during the week, on game weekends he drinks excessively, often to the point of passing out. Other research has found that when comparing same-age peers, those enrolled in college tend to drink in a riskier fashion than those who are not enrolled in college (Timberlake et al., 2007).

The age and gender of college students affects their drinking patterns. Specifically, Likis-Werle and Borders (2017) found that 18- and 19-year-old students drank as much as they could at each sitting, but older students had more responsibilities, so their frequency and quantity of drinking decreased. The researchers concluded that younger students were not able to regulate their drinking as much as older students.

Drinking may lead to behavior that one regrets. One study found that 35% of female college drinkers reported regretting a sexual situation after drinking, 23% failed to use birth control or protect from sexually transmitted infections, and 22% had sex with someone they would not ordinarily have sex with (Moorer et al., 2013). Risks for women and men drinking excessive amounts of alcohol include substance-related sexual assault as well as unplanned sexual activity (see Chapter 10).

Chapter 10 discussed posttraumatic stress disorder (PTSD), a condition that can result after a traumatic event. Much research has shown a relationship between drinking alcohol and PTSD, namely that those who have PTSD may use alcohol as a coping mechanism (Valenstein-Mah et al., 2019). One theory is that students use substances to self-medicate, as a way to avoid or cope with negative thoughts and feelings that are a result of the trauma. Read et al. (2012) found that risk for problem substance use is greatest for those with PTSD at the beginning of the academic year. The transition to college is a particularly difficult time, and the risk for those who enter college with past traumatic experiences (that result in PTSD) are at heightened risk of substance abuse.

While alcohol may be among the most commonly used drugs in college, many other substances have gained popularity among college students. See Table 12.1 for a list of commonly abused substances.

Table 12.1

Drug Categories, Common Names, and Their Effects

Drug category	Type of drugs	Common names	Effects of intoxication
Sedative-hypnotics (depressants)	alcohol, barbiturates (Seconol, Qualuudes), tranquilizers (Valium, Librium, Ativan, Xanax)	Booze, barbs, ludes, tranks, bisquits	Drowsiness, slows CNS, confusion, uncoordinated movements
Stimulants	cocaine, meth-amphetamines, amphetamines, caffeine, nicotine	C, coke, flake, crack, meth, crystal, crank, black beauty, java, joe	Talkativeness, alertness, stimulates CNS, paranoia, increase in anxiety, decrease in appetite, hyperactivity
Cannabinols	marijuana, hash, hash oil	Pot, dope, weed, hash, sheesh, herb, doobie	Decrease in motivation, red eyes, decrease in motor skill ability, increase in hunger, excessive laughing, paranoia
Opioids	heroin, Demerol, Diluadid, morphine, codeine, Percodan, methadone, opium	Junk, smack, oxy, China, white, H, horse	Nausea, nodding out, vomiting, watery eyes and nose, insensitivity to pain, detached
Hallucinogens	LSD, mescaline, PCP, MDMA, peyote	Sid, ex, rocket fuel	Impaired judgement, hallucinations, change in perception
Inhalants	gasoline, aerosols, glue, liquid paper, nitrous oxide	Whippets, nitros, rush	Dizziness, odor of chemicals, severe headaches, blackouts, hallucinations

Note. Adapted from *A Contemporary Approach to Substance Abuse and Addiction Counseling (2nd ed.)*, by F. Brooks and B. McHenry, 2015, p. 41. Copyright © 2015 by the American Counseling Association. Adapted with permission.

Marijuana

There is likely no drug as controversial as marijuana. Its medicinal effects have been substantiated, and many states allow its use in certain conditions. As recreational marijuana use is legalized in some states, use among undergraduate students is rising (Bae & Kerr, 2019) and may affect use of other substances. In fact, Alley et al. (2020)

found that for students ages 21 years and over, binge drinking decreased following the legalization of marijuana for recreation, whereas for those under 21, sedative misuse increased. There is also a fallacy that using marijuana is not as hazardous as using other drugs, in part due to the lack of a withdrawal syndrome. Marijuana affects one's memory, learning, perception, concentration, judgment, and physical coordination (National Institute on Drug Abuse, 2019). ACHA (2022) found that approximately 23% of college students (male and female) reported using marijuana in the last 3 months. Using marijuana negatively affects students' grade point averages (Martinez et al., 2015).

Stimulants

Stimulants (e.g., Ritalin, Adderall) are primarily used in the treatment of attention deficit hyperactivity disorder, although they are commonly used and abused by college students who do not have this condition. The misuse of stimulants by college students appears to be strongly motivated by the desire to improve academic performance (Benson et al., 2015). Students take these drugs hoping to stay awake longer, concentrate on studying, increase alertness, and ultimately improve their grades. This was Hannah's strategy to studying when she was feeling out of time due to swimming practice. Benson et al. (2015) found that overwhelmingly students who misused stimulants tended to be Caucasian, male, part of a Greek-letter organization, and have a lower GPA than nonusers. Nonprescription stimulants were used about equally by male and female students and correlated with past 30-day marijuana and tobacco use (Fairman et al., 2020). These students tended to stay awake longer and party longer than those who had prescriptions for such medication, which indicates recreational uses of the drugs. Students who use stimulants without a prescription are likely to get the drugs from students who have prescriptions. It seems many students believe that stimulant use will lead to better grades. Research has found that students who believe in the academic benefits of nonprescription stimulant use are more likely to use them and also tend to drink alcohol and use marijuana more frequently than students who do not believe in the benefits of stimulant use (Arria et al., 2018). Interestingly, students' beliefs about stimulant use and improved academic performance are in stark contrast to what science has shown, which is that no academic advantage or benefit exists (Arria et al., 2017). Along with the desire to achieve academically, some college students abuse stimulants to lose weight, since the drugs also function as an appetite suppressant (Ward et al., 2016).

Opioids

National data suggest that the misuse of prescription opioids among 18- to 24-year-olds is proportionally higher than other age groups (Hughes et al., 2016; SAMHSA, 2019). Further, college students have reported prescription opioid misuse as a means of self-medicating depression and other emotional distress (Kenne et al., 2017; Lord et al., 2011). In a study by Davis et al. (2020), more than 21% of college students reported prescription opioid use over the last 12 months. Another alarming statistic from this study is that 40% reported suicidal ideation, believed to be associated with drug use. Specifically, those reporting prescription opioid misuse were significantly more likely to report suicidal thoughts, plans, and attempts. While prescription opioid misuse is understood to be used by students to manage negative mood states, the initial euphoria experienced is quickly replaced by recurrent depressive feelings and thoughts. Students who use opioids are likely to isolate from friends and family, furthering their feelings of loneliness, which only fuels their feelings of depression. Professionals must keep in mind that use of opioids is likely associated with underlying psychological distress.

Multiple Substance Use

Many college students don't limit themselves to the use of only one drug. Higher education professionals need to be aware that use of one substance does not necessarily preclude using others. More than half (59%) of 4-year college students who drank alcohol in the past year reported using marijuana and alcohol at the same time and being drunk and high at the same time (Patrick et al., 2018). Davis et al. (2020) found that approximately half (48%) of their sample of college students reported marijuana use and more than 70% engaged in binge drinking over the same 12-month period. A wealth of research cites the consequences and deleterious outcomes of using marijuana and alcohol together. These include more car accidents, social consequences (e.g., saying or doing embarrassing things), mental health problems, dependence symptoms, vomiting, increased risk of blackouts, and increased likelihood of unprotected sex (Jackson et al., 2020). Alcohol and marijuana use have been linked to poor academic performance (Arria et al., 2015; Hingson & White, 2013; White & Hingson, 2013). Some students may receive disciplinary action for their substance use for violating the school's alcohol or drug policies. Research has found that some decrease in students' drinking may occur as a result of getting caught (Terlecki et al., 2015), but the extent to which the decreases are maintained is unknown. Students who are disciplined usually represent those who are heavy drinkers.

All substance abuse disorders are considered on a continuum of mild, moderate, and severe. In the *Diagnostic and Statistical Manual of Mental Disorders, Fifth Edition (DSM-5)*, the American Psychiatric Association (APA, 2013) set criteria for substance abuse disorders, which are applicable to almost all substances. The number of criteria an individual displays dictates the severity. Some of the criteria include having to take more and more of the substance to achieve the same effect, using larger amounts for longer periods of time than intended, and intense desire for the substance. An example of these criteria is the student who repeatedly goes out intending to have only two beers and ends up staying out all night. Other criteria include excessive time spent securing, using, and then recovering from the drug; unsuccessful efforts to cut back on use; and withdrawal symptoms. This might be the student who vows *every* Monday morning to not drink again and by Thursday finds themselves at a fraternity party getting drunk. The *DSM-5* notes that as a general rule a mild condition is considered two or three criteria, moderate is four or five criteria, and severe is six or more criteria (APA, 2013). Students may not be doing well at work or school, they may give up socializing with those who do not use substances, and they may pull back from family and friends (APA, 2013). In some cases, students use the substance in situations that are risky or hazardous. Driving while under the influence is a good example of this criterion. Essentially, someone who has a problem with a substance continues to use the drug despite significant problems related to the drug or impairments in their daily functioning. A common example here is the student who begins to fail classes but continues to use drugs. Research has found marijuana use and other illicit drug use were significantly related to discontinuous enrollment in college, but the same was not true for alcohol use disorder (Arria et al., 2013).

Approaching the Issue With Students

Burke et al. (2017) stated that the higher education professional may be a student's initial point of contact regarding their substance abuse and are in a unique position to influence the trajectory of the institutional response to the student's situation. As a higher education professional, you will want to discern the student's level of use but also approach the issue in a way that does not sound judgmental, blaming, or "parental." But, given the risk of overdose when using substances, all reports of excessive substance abuse should be taken seriously.

Knowing the signs of substance abuse will aid in identifying a problem with a student. Be careful not to recommend "stopping immediately" if you are not trained to determine the level of substance dependence. For example, if a student has developed a dependence on alcohol, stopping suddenly can lead to seizures. Giving up substances requires guidance by a mental health professional or substance abuse counselor.

Many students, and others, who use alcohol often minimize their use, so approaching the subject can be tricky. They often report using much less than they actually do. Some may even be hostile when you approach the issue of excessive use. Understanding that students, like most substance users, are likely to underestimate their use of substances will help you avoid frustration when asking students about their substance use. Students may engage in minimizing ("It was only five beers"), rationalizing ("Everyone at the party was doing it"), or denial ("I did not even touch that stuff"). This makes evaluation difficult. As discussed in Chapter 2, avoiding the use of "why" questions with students who are exhibiting substance abuse problems is advised. "Why did you drink that much?" or "Why would you smoke dope?" comes across as judgmental and is likely to yield a defensive response from the student. You are likely to get more information by saying, "So tell me a bit about what happened at the party" or, "Sounds like you had quite a weekend. What do you remember?"

You may find it difficult to offer empathy when you think the student is being dishonest with you about substance use. Remember that denial is a coping mechanism that helps some students and is often occurring on an unconscious basis (Miller & Carrol, 2010). Recognize that the student may not be sharing an objective reality but rather their view of the situation. It may also be difficult to be accepting of some of the behavior that you hear from a student, such as driving under the influence, using illegal drugs, or pressuring others to drink (e.g., hazing in Greek-letter organizations). What would it be like for you to listen to a student describing a drunk driving incident if one of your family members had been the victim of a drunk driver? As difficult as it may be, you must set aside your values and experiences, be nonjudgmental, and focus on the student in front of you. Remember, their engaging in this behavior is not about you—it is about them.

There is a simple screening method for alcohol use called the CAGE (Ewing, 1984). It consists of four questions that follow the acronym: "Have you ever felt a need to **c**ut down on your drinking?" "Have you ever felt **a**ngry or annoyed at someone because they commented that your drank too much?" "Have you ever felt bad or **g**uilty because you drank too much?" and "Have you ever had a drink first thing in the morning to steady your nerves and get rid of a hangover (**e**ye opener)?" A positive response to any of these questions can indicate a problem with alcohol. While you may not want to formally ask these questions of a student, the questions can help serve as a guide in a discussion about problematic alcohol use.

Inquiring about when a student first began to use substances can be helpful in understanding their pattern of use. Likis-Werle (2020) reported that a younger age of exposure correlates with a higher risk of dependency. Using regularly before the age of 15 exponentially increases the likelihood of developing a substance addiction. As stated before, some substance use by students is experimental or done only in certain situations (e.g., at games or parties), while other students come to college with a preexisting substance use issue. It is important to note that frequency alone does not predict problematic use. For example, a student may use only at fraternity parties but then uses to excess and engages in risky behavior.

When and How to Make a Referral to Counseling

The student with a substance abuse issue may demonstrate ambivalence about change, and the higher education professional needs to be accepting. There may be times the student is very honest about the problems that using drugs causes, and at other times they may be unwilling to admit there is a problem. Leaving the world of substance abuse for a lifestyle of abstinence and recovery can seem overwhelming to anyone entering recovery, but perhaps more so to young students who have a whole life ahead of them. As Lewis et al. (2019) stated, "Empathy can help clients take the important step of openly examining their feelings about both the positive and negative aspects of drug use" (p. 110). Since most treatment programs advocate for abstinence, imagine how difficult it must be for a 19-year-old student to think about never having another drink for the rest of their life. Given the potential lethality of some substances, higher education professionals will need to be thorough in their understanding of the student's use.

Confrontation should be avoided when addressing someone with a substance abuse disorder. When a student presents as defensive and resistant, do not push them but, rather, explain the choice available to them: "You don't have to seek help now. You can continue to use and perhaps handle things differently. It is your choice." Giving the student choices or exploring these choices shows respect for the student and lets them know you are there to listen without judgment. This leaves the door open for them to come to you should things escalate or when they are ready to admit they need help.

There are a range of options for substance abuse treatment, and the choice will depend on the severity of each student's use, dependence, and current functioning. Levels of care include centers where detoxification from the substance can occur and stabilization can begin. These centers are typically short-term residential facilities that operate under medical supervision. This type of treatment would be necessary for students who have severe alcohol problems. Outpatient treatment (not requiring overnight stays) occurs on a continuum of care from partial hospitalization (spending most of the day at a facility and returning home at night) to weekly meetings with a mental health professional who is trained in addictions counseling. Learn about local centers and agencies that work with students in order to make an appropriate referral for services. For example, the higher education professional could say, "Lorena, given what you told me about drinking the past few weeks and how it has gotten out of control, I was wondering if you might want to talk to someone else about it?" Being aware of your institution and department protocols is also critical to knowing what steps to take.

One recommendation to students who may be thinking about cutting back or stopping their substance use is a 12-step program. The use of 12-step and other self-help programs (e.g., Alcoholics Anonymous, Narcotics Anonymous) has been very helpful for people with substance disorders. The programs are free, open to anyone, and exist all around the world, likely including on your college campus. Alcoholics Anonymous groups for LGBTQIA+ students are common too. Operating as a social support system for recovery, the groups are not led by professionals but by others who are also in recovery. Recommending to a student that they try out a group on campus may be a helpful first step since these groups have little formal structure and may help students connect with others in a similar situation. You might say, "Quinn, have you heard about Alcoholics Anonymous? Based on some of what you told me about your father drinking heavily and you starting to have some concerns, maybe you could check out a meeting? It's free and here on campus on Tuesday nights. There is no commitment. What do you think?"

For students who wish to get treatment yet stay in college, it may be difficult to find the right balance. The Haven is a treatment facility that partners with universities across the United States to offer housing and other support to students in recovery. Haven Sober Living Residences are student-led, clinically supervised houses and apartments where peers in recovery help each other navigate sobriety while enjoying the company of their peers.

Approaching the student with genuine care and concern, and not condescension, will help with referral. Letting the student know that you are genuinely worried about them may make them more open to treatment recommendations. Whatever recommendation you provide to the student, be sure to remain positive in your outlook. Reminding the student that there are many professionals and agencies that are equipped to help them can provide hope. Also, explaining to the student that many others struggle with the same issue, and that they don't have to do it alone, can help the student overcome any feelings of trepidation as they embark on change.

Conclusion

Substance use by college students is an ongoing concern for higher education professionals. The newfound freedom of being away from home with few restrictions and peer influence can contribute to substance use by some college students, while others may enter college with preexisting drug or alcohol problems. There is a range of substances that college students commonly use, including alcohol, marijuana, and stimulants. Higher education professionals will need to distinguish recreational or social use from more chronic, problematic use. Approaching students whose substance use is of concern is a tricky process; it is important to show concern without judgment. Recognizing that the student may also under report their use is critical in determining if a problematic pattern of behavior is present. Fortunately, many resources exist, and higher education professionals are well situated to make referrals. Programs to assist students include self-help, outpatient, and residential centers. Connecting students to interventions most appropriate for them is the first step in the help and recovery process.

References

Alley, Z. M., Kerr, D. C., & Bae, H. (2020). Trends in college students' alcohol, nicotine, prescription opioid and other drug use after recreational marijuana legalization: 2008–2018. *Addictive Behaviors, 102*, 1–7. https://doi.org/10.1016/j.addbeh.2019.106212

American College Health Association. (2022). *American College Health Association— National college health assessment III: Undergraduate student reference group executive summary fall 2021.* https://www.acha.org/documents/ncha/NCHA-III_FALL_2021_UNDERGRADUATE_REFERENCE_GROUP_EXECUTIVE_SUMMARY.pdf

American Psychiatric Association. (2013). *Diagnostic and statistical manual of mental disorders* (5th ed.).

Arria, A. M., Caldeira, K. M., Allen, H. K., Bugbee, B. A., Vincent, K. B., & O'Grady, K. E. (2017). Prevalence and incidence of drug use among college students: An 8-year longitudinal analysis. *The American Journal of Drug and Alcohol Abuse, 43*(6), 711–718. https://doi.org/10.1080/00952990.2017.1310219

Arria, A. M., Caldeira, K. M., Bugbee, B. A., Vincent, K. B., & O'Grady, K. E. (2015). The academic consequences of marijuana use during college. *Psychology of Addictive Behaviors, 29*(3), 564–567. https//doi.org/10.1037/adb0000108

Arria, A. M., Garnier-Dykstra, L. M., Caldeira, K. M., Vincent, K. B., Winick, E. R., & O'Grady, K. E. (2013). Drug use patterns and continuous enrollment in college: Results from a longitudinal study. *Journal of Studies on Alcohol and Drugs, 74*(1), 71–83. https://doi.org/10.15288/jsad.2013.74.71

Arria, A. M., Geisner, I. M., Cimini, M. D., Kilmer, J. R., Caldeira, K. M., Barrall, A. L., Vincent, K. B., Fossos-Wong, N., Yeh, J.-C., Rhew, I., Lee, C. M., Subramaniam, G. A., Liu, D., & Larimer, M. E. (2018). Perceived academic benefit is associated with nonmedical prescription stimulant use among college students. *Addictive Behaviors, 76*, 27–33. https://doi.org/10.1016/j.addbeh.2017.07.013

Bae, H., & Kerr, D. C. (2019). Marijuana use trends among college students in states with and without legalization of recreational use: Initial and longer-term changes from 2008 to 2018. *Addiction, 115*(6), 1115–1124. https://doi.org/10.1111/add.14939

Benson, K., Flory, K., Humphreys, K. L., & Lee, S. S. (2015). Misuse of stimulant medication among college students: A comprehensive review and meta-analysis. *Clinical Child and Family Psychology Review, 18*(1), 50–76. https://doi.org/10.1007/s10567-014-0177-z

Borsari, B., Murphy, J. G., & Barnett, N. P. (2007). Predictors of alcohol use during the first year of college: Implications for prevention. *Addictive Behaviors, 32*(10), 2062–2086. https://dx.doi.org/10.1016%2Fj.addbeh.2007.01.017

Buckman, J. F., Farris, S. G., & Yusko, D. A. (2013). A national study of substance use behaviors among NCAA male athletes who use banned performance enhancing substances. *Drug and Alcohol Dependence, 131*(1–2), 50–55. https://doi.org/10.1016/j.drugalcdep.2013.04.023

Burke, M. G., Sauerheber, J. D., Hughey, A. W., & Laves, K. S. (2017). *Helping skills for working with college students: Applying counseling theory to student affairs practice.* Routledge.

Davis, R. E., Doyle, N. A., & Nahar, V. K. (2020). Association between prescription opioid misuse and dimensions of suicidality among college students. *Psychiatry Research, 287*, 1–6. https://doi.org/10.1016/j.psychres.2019.07.002

Donohue, B., Loughran, T., Pitts, M., Gavrilova, Y., Chow, G. M., Soto-Nevarez, A., & Schubert, K. (2016). Preliminary development of a brief intervention to prevent alcohol misuse and enhance sport performance in collegiate athletes. *Journal of Drug Abuse, 2*(3), 1–9. https://doi.org/10.21767/2471-853X.100035

Druckman, J. N., Gilli, M., Klar, S., & Robison, J. (2015). Measuring drug and alcohol use among college student-athletes. *Social Science Quarterly, 96*(2), 369–380. https://doi.org/10.1111/ssqu.12135

Essig Aberg, S., Adler, A., Liu, J., & Zuckerman, D. (n.d.). *"Study drug" abuse by college students: What you need to know*. National Center for Health Research. http://www.center4research.org/study-drug-abuse-college-students

Ewing, J. A. (1984). Detecting alcoholism: The CAGE questionnaire. *Journal of the American Medical Association, 252*(14), 1905–1907. https://doi.org/10.1001/jama.1984.03350140051025

Fairman, R. T., Vu, M., Haardörfer, R., Windle, M., & Berg, C. J. (2020). Prescription stimulant use among young adult college students: Who uses, why, and what are the consequences? *Journal of American College Health, 69*(7), 1–8. https://doi.org/10.1080/07448481.2019.1706539

Grossbard, J. R., Mastroleo, N. R., Geisner, I. M., Atkins, D., Ray, A. E., Kilmer, J. R., Mallett, K., Larimer, M. E., & Turrisi, R. (2016). Drinking norms, readiness to change, and gender as moderators of a combined alcohol intervention for first-year college students. *Addictive Behaviors, 52*, 75–82. https://doi.org/10.1016/j.addbeh.2015.07.028

Hingson, R. W., & White, A. (2013). Trends in extreme binge drinking among U.S. high school seniors. *Pediatrics, 167*(11), 996–998. https://doi.org/10.1001/jamapediatrics.2013.3083

Hughes, A., Williams, M. R., Lipari, R. N., Bose, J., Copello, E. A. P., & Kroutil, L. A. (2016). Prescription drug use and misuse in the United States: Results from the 2015 National Survey on Drug Use and Health. *NSDUH Data Review*, A1–A24.

Jackson, K. M., Sokolovsky, A. W., Gunn, R. L., & White, H. R. (2020). Consequences of alcohol and marijuana use among college students: Prevalence rates and attributions to substance-specific versus simultaneous use. *Psychology of Addictive Behaviors, 34*(2), 370–381. https://doi.org/10.1037/adb0000545

Kenne, D. R., Fischbein, R. L., Tan, A. S., & Banks, M. (2017). The use of substances other than nicotine in electronic cigarettes among college students. *Substance Abuse: Research and Treatment, 11*, 1–8. https://doi.org/10.1177/1178221817733736

Kerr, D. L., Ding, K., & Chaya, J. (2014). Substance use of lesbian, gay, bisexual and heterosexual college students. *American Journal of Health Behavior, 38*(6), 951–962. https://doi.org/10.5993/ajhb.38.6.17

Lewis, J. A., Dana, R. Q., & Blevins, G. A. (2019). *Substance abuse counseling* (6th ed.). Cengage Learning.

Lewis, T. (2015). Alcohol addiction. In R. Smith (Ed.), *Treatment strategies for substance and process addictions* (pp. 33–56). American Counseling Association.

Likis-Werle, E. (2020). Substance use and addiction. In D. A. Paladino, L. M. Gonzalez, & J. C. Watson (Eds.), *College counseling and student development: Theory, practice and campus collaboration* (pp. 317–329). American Counseling Association.

Likis-Werle, E., & Borders, L. D. (2017). College women's experiences and perceptions of drinking: A phenomenological exploration. *Journal of College Counseling, 20*(2), 99–112. https://doi.org/10.1002/JOCC.12063

Lord, S., Brevard, J., & Budman, S. (2011). Connecting to young adults: An online social network survey of beliefs and attitudes associated with prescription opioid misuse among college students. *Substance Use & Misuse, 46*(1), 66–76. https://doi.org/10.3109/10826084.2011.521371

Manning, P., Pring, L., & Glider, P. (2012). Relevance of campus climate for alcohol and other drug use among LGBTQ community college students: A statewide qualitative assessment. *Community College Journal of Research and Practice, 36*(7), 494–503. https://doi.org/10.1080/10668926.2012.664088

Martinez, J. A., Roth, M. G., Johnson, D. N., & Jones, J. A. (2015). How robustly does cannabis use associate to college grades? Findings from two cohorts. *Journal of Drug Education, 45*(1), 56–67. https://doi.org/10.1177%2F0047237915596606

Marzell, M., Bavarian, N., Paschall, M. J., Mair, C., & Saltz, R. F. (2015). Party characteristics, drinking settings, and college students' risk of intoxication: A multi-campus study. *The Journal of Primary Prevention, 36*(4), 247–258. https://doi.org/10.1007/s10935-015-0393-4

McCabe, S. E., Veliz, P., & Schulenberg, J. E. (2018). How collegiate fraternity and sorority involvement relates to substance use during young adulthood and substance use disorders in early midlife: A national longitudinal study. *Journal of Adolescent Health*, *62*(3), S35–S43. https://doi.org/10.1016/j.jadohealth.2017.09.029

Miller, W., & Carroll, K. (2010). *Rethinking substance abuse: What the science shows, and what we should do about it*. The Guilford Press.

Moorer, K. D., Madson, M. B., Mohn, R. S., & Nicholson, B. C. (2013). Alcohol consumption and negative sex-related consequences among college women: The moderating role of alcohol protective behavioral strategies. *Journal of Drug Education*, *43*, 365–383. https://doi.org/10.2190/DE.43.4.e

National Collegiate Athletic Association. (2018). *NCAA student-athlete substance use study: Executive summary June 2018*. https://ncaaorg.s3.amazonaws.com/research/substance/2017RES_SubstanceUseExecutiveSummary.pdf

National Collegiate Athletic Association. (2021). *Drug-testing program*. https://ncaaorg.s3.amazonaws.com/ssi/substance/2021-22/2021-22SSI_DrugTestingProgram.pdf

National Institute on Alcohol Abuse and Alcoholism. (2020). *College drinking*. https://www.niaaa.nih.gov/publications/brochures-and-fact-sheets/college-drinking

National Institute on Drug Abuse. (2019). *Drug facts*. https://www.drugabuse.gov/sites/default/files/drugfacts-marijuana.pdf

National Institute on Drug Abuse. (2020). *Drugs, brain, and behavior: The science of addiction*. https://www.drugabuse.gov/sites/default/files/soa.pdf

Patrick, M. E., Fairlie, A. M., & Lee, C. M. (2018). Motives for simultaneous alcohol and marijuana use among young adults. *Addictive Behaviors*, *76*, 363–369. https://doi.org/10.1016/j.addbeh.2017.08.027

Read, J. P., Colder, C. R., Merrill, J. E., Ouimette, P., White, J., & Swartout, A. (2012). Trauma and posttraumatic stress symptoms predict alcohol and other drug consequence trajectories in the first year of college. *Journal of Consulting and Clinical Psychology*, *80*(3), 426–439. https://doi.org/10.1037/a0028210

Reed, E., Prado, G., Matsumoto, A., & Amaro, H. (2010). Alcohol and drug use and related consequences among gay, lesbian and bisexual college students: Role of experiencing violence, feeling safe on campus, and perceived stress. *Addictive Behaviors*, *35*(2), 168–171. https://doi.org/10.1016/j.addbeh.2009.09.005

Reetz, D. R., Bershad, C., LeViness, P., & Whitlock, M. (2016). *The Association for University and College Counseling Center Directors annual survey*. Association for University and College Counseling Center Directors. https://www.aucccd.org/assets/documents/aucccd%202016%20monograph%20-%20public.pdf

Substance Abuse and Mental Health Services Administration. (2019). *Results from the 2018 national survey on drug use and health: Detailed tables*. https://www.samhsa.gov/data/sites/default/files/cbhsq-reports/NSDUHDetailedTabs2018R2/NSDUHDetailedTabs2018.pdf

Substance Abuse and Mental Health Services Administration. (2021, March). *Facts on college student drinking*. https://store.samhsa.gov/sites/default/files/SAMHSA_Digital_Download/PEP21-03-10-006.pdf

Terlecki, M. A., Buckner, J. D., Larimer, M. E., & Copeland, A. L. (2015). Randomized controlled trial of brief alcohol screening and intervention for college students for heavy-drinking mandated and volunteer undergraduates: 12-month outcomes. *Psychology of Addictive Behaviors*, *29*(1), 2–16. https://doi.org/10.1037/adb0000056

Timberlake, D. S., Hopfer, C. J., Rhee, S. H., Friedman, N. P., Haberstick, B. C., Lessem, J. M., & Hewitt, J. K. (2007). College attendance and its effect on drinking behaviors in a longitudinal study of adolescents. *Alcoholism: Clinical and Experimental Research*, *31*(6), 1020–1030. https://doi.org/10.1111/j.1530-0277.2007.00383.x

Tremblay, P. F., Graham, K., Wells, S., Harris, R., Pulford, R., & Roberts, S. (2010). When do first-year college students drink most during the academic year? An internet-based study of daily and weekly drinking. *Journal of American College Health, 58*(5), 401–411. https://doi.org/10.1080/07448480903540465

Valenstein-Mah, H., Simpson, T. L., Bowen, S., Enkema, M. C., Bird, E. R., Cho, H. I., & Larimer, M. E. (2019). Feasibility pilot of a brief mindfulness intervention for college students with posttraumatic stress symptoms and problem drinking. *Mindfulness, 10*(7), 1255–1268. https://doi.org/10.1007/s12671-018-1077-y

Ward, R. M., Oswald, B. B., & Galante, M. (2016). Prescription stimulant misuse, alcohol abuse, and disordered eating among college students. *Journal of Alcohol and Drug Education, 60*(1), 59–80. https://search.proquest.com/docview/1802191631?accountid=6724

White, A., & Hingson, R. (2013). The burden of alcohol use: Excessive alcohol consumption and related consequences among college students. *Alcohol Research: Current Reviews, 35*(2), 201–218. https://www.ncbi.nlm.nih.gov/pmc/articles/PMC3908712/pdf/arcr-35-2-201.pdf

CHAPTER 13

Grief and Loss

During college, many students will experience some form of loss. It might be the death of a friend or relative. They will begin to feel a deep sense of grief and sadness. Knowing how to identify students going through grief and loss, and when and how to intervene, is important for higher education professionals to help students navigate these difficult situations. Many students have never experienced loss before, and their first exposure to this type of grief can be paralyzing for them. This chapter will help orient higher education professionals to the grief process and how to get students the assistance and support they need.

Basic Signs and Symptoms of Grief and Loss

Research shows that about 1 in 3 college students has lost a family member or close friend within the last 12 months; this same statistic holds true for all young adults ages 18 to 25 years (HealGrief, n.d.). Not only might they experience their own loss of a loved one, but the overall mortality rates on campus support the assertion that students are likely to be impacted by death, either directly or proximal. It's not surprising, therefore, that an estimated 22% to 30% of all college students will be affected by death at some point in their college careers (Balk, 2008). In 2014, an estimated 108,000 full-time college students reported a suicide attempt in the previous year (National Action Alliance for Suicide Prevention and the Research Prioritization Task Force, 2014). Suicide is the second leading of cause of death among traditional-aged college students (Centers for Disease Control and Prevention, 2020). In a study by Frazier et al. (2009), 47% of participants reported that an unexpected death was the most traumatic event experienced during their college years.

Although losses may be difficult to handle at any time, college students typically live away from home, without the support of family, which may exacerbate feelings of bereavement. Not only do these students suffer a loss, they also often feel as if they cannot take the time needed to grieve properly without somehow letting others down or falling behind in their studies. They often have obligations, both in and out of the classroom, and feel that by taking the needed "time out" for themselves to process the loss, they will in turn fail to honor their commitments. So, they often push their feelings aside and fail to deal with them. And when these students do not cope with their grief, both their mental and their physical health can be affected.

Everyone experiences grief differently; there is no "right" way to grieve. Higher education professionals may find it helpful to know the stages of grief and how to intervene with students who have experienced a significant loss. It is also important for professionals to be able to distinguish the grief process from a prolonged depression. Some students will tackle their grief head-on, with lots of expressions of emotion and sadness; others will not want to handle it all, pushing their grief aside.

Grief and Loss

Case Study

Julia is a sophomore in college. She's had a good experience so far and is well connected on campus. She is a member of many campus organizations, including a sorority, club volleyball, and alternative spring break. Her campus is about a 5-hour drive from her home. She comes from a close family. In the summer before her sophomore year, Julia's grandmother's health began to deteriorate. Though Julia was hesitant to return to school, her parents and younger brother assured her that it was in her best interest to continue her studies. She had long talks with her grandmother and made the difficult decision to return to campus in the fall. That semester was challenging for Julia because she felt the constant pull of home. She worried about her grandmother and wanted to be there for her family. In October, her grandmother took a turn for the worse. After speaking with her academic advisor and professors, Julia decided to go home. While there, her grandmother passed away.

After a few weeks at home, Julia returns to campus. She struggles with adjusting back to life on campus, especially having missed so many classes and so much time with her friends. Julia is sad, misses her family, and has trouble concentrating on her classes. She often experiences mood swings. Her friends want to help, but they don't know what to say or how to support her. She is close to some faculty members as well as her sorority advisor; all of them want to help her during this very emotional time.

According to the foundational work of Kübler-Ross (1969), there are five stages of grief and loss. Not everyone will experience these stages in the same way, or in the same order; however, most people will go through these stages at some point during their grieving process. The five stages are as follows:

1. **Denial.** During this stage, people *believe* that their loved one has died, but they have trouble *accepting* that they have lost this person. In the case of Julia, it might be very easy for her to remain in this stage—she is away from home and does not need to confront the loss directly. She can easily return to her life in college and act almost as if her grandmother is simply back at home.
2. **Anger.** In the anger stage, people become upset at the deceased or at themselves for not preventing their loved one's death. Reaching this stage is important, as it allows the grieving individual to start healing (Bolden, 2007). In this stage, Julia might act out in anger toward her friends or classmates; they might notice her mood change or her temper shorten.
3. **Bargaining.** During this stage, people begin to ask "what if" and ponder "if only." They question whether they could have done anything differently to prevent the loss of their loved one. For Julia, she might regret her decision to return to college after the summer, questioning whether that decision in any way influenced the loss. She may experience feelings of guilt and regret over her choice.
4. **Depression.** This is a very normal stage in the grieving process; in fact, feelings of depression and sadness are necessary for healing. In the case study, Julia is sad, misses her family, and has trouble concentrating on her classes.
5. **Acceptance.** At this point, the person can accept the loss and find a way to move on. For Julia, she will benefit from the empathy and support of others, knowing she is away from her family and loved ones.

Understanding these stages will help higher education professionals to support grieving students. Keep in mind: Not everyone will experience all these stages in the same order, and they may go back and forth between the stages. Professionals should also consider educating students on these stages so they can empathize with their peers and know that these reactions are normal.

Approaching the Issue With Students

It is essential that higher education professionals support college students who are grieving; these students are not receiving the support structure they might be getting if they were at home. Not only is it likely they have never experienced a loved one's death, but they are probably living away from home for the first time. Although they may be surrounded by friends, their peers might not understand grief and thus be unable to show the empathy and support so needed during this difficult time (HealGrief, n.d.). Counseling centers already face considerable demands, and grieving students are at high risk for many concerning issues such as feelings of isolation, an inability to focus, a lack of energy, and depression. If these students do not get the support they need, such problems could escalate to dropping out of school, increased depression, and perhaps even suicide.

Grieving college students are at greater risk than their peers for a host of physical, academic, social, developmental, and emotional issues (Balk, 2008; Servaty-Seib & Hamilton, 2006). Students who have suffered a significant loss report feeling alone, helpless, unsupported, and like no one "gets it" (Fajgenbaum et al., 2012). While they are grieving, these students sit by as their peers continue with normal college life. As their friends continue to attend parties and social gatherings without them, this sense of isolation can continue and intensify.

Research shows that grieving people rarely seek help (Balk, 2008). Although some grieving students might choose to see a therapist, most will not see bereavement as a reason to attend counseling. All grieving students, however, are facing the same issues. Julia's case is very common and highlights the physical, behavioral, interpersonal, academic, and emotional toll that can take place.

Physical

Mourning often has physical side effects (Balk & Vesta, 1998; Hardison et al., 2005; King, 1998; Oltjenbruns, 1996). Problems sleeping—and insomnia in particular—are common. Grieving students report a higher level of insomnia and disrupted sleep patterns (Hardison et al., 2005). Sleep deprivation leads to many additional harms, as it drains energy from other areas of life. Grieving students can lack the physical energy needed to tackle daily tasks such as simply attending class. This fatigue can compound an already difficult situation.

Behavioral

Grieving students often lack focus and find it tough to stay on task (Balk et al., 1993; Balk & Vesta, 1998). Managing time and meeting deadlines can be a challenge for many college students; for those who are grieving, it is often exacerbated by sleep deprivation and other coexisting factors.

Interpersonal

As in Julia's case, friends often do not know how to help. As a result, they sometimes minimize the situation and dismiss the emotions of the bereaved. If they have not experienced a loss themselves, they may not understand why their friend cannot just "move on." They also fear not knowing what to say—and may avoid their grieving friend out of fear of saying the wrong thing. This avoidance can lead to further isolation for the student. At times, friends might find a person's ongoing grief both hard to handle as a supportive friend and might find it impacting them personally as well. Consequently, they end up pulling away from the griever (Balk & Vesta, 1998; Oltjenbruns, 1996).

Academic

Students must focus on their classes and meet their academic expectations while in college. Because this obligation becomes increasingly difficult for a grieving student to manage, academic struggles will probably be the most obvious sign to a higher education professional that something is wrong. One of the first areas affected will be class attendance, grades, and persistence; grades often drop significantly in the first semester following a loss (Servaty-Seib & Hamilton, 2006). Though not necessarily more important than other aspects of life, such academic concerns are time sensitive and will most likely require immediate intervention.

Emotional

Grieving affects everyone differently. Grieving students may burst into tears for no reason, and with no obvious trigger. They might be sitting in class, and something might strike a chord, prompting an emotional response. Often those nearby do not know how best to respond to these emotional episodes. If they have experienced other losses in their life, this most recent loss may remind them of other losses from their past.

As higher education professionals, we must find out what students need and how to help them. Our role is to intervene individually and assist wherever possible. We know that it is unlikely that a student grieving will seek support from the counseling center, but instead of leaving bereaved students to handle their grief on their own—assuming that, in time, they will work through the grieving process—we should try to determine what interventions can be put in place to help them avoid disrupting their academic path (Balk, 2008; Servaty-Seib & Hamilton, 2006).

Often bereaved students begin to question what has meaning in their lives. College and academics can sometimes feel less important after losing someone significant. One participant in a study by Cupit et al. (2016) commented that her grades no longer had the same level of significance. She had become more focused on her friends and family and spending time on what made her the happiest. When higher education professionals talk with students after a loss, they should find ways to connect meaning to the college experience. Furthermore, students who have suffered a loss need flexibility with their academic work and deadlines (Culpit et al., 2016). It would be particularly helpful to show empathy and understanding for these students in terms of flexibility and sensitivity related to their academic pressures and demands. Recognize this can be helpful for both faculty and staff as they converse with students and work together to help them succeed in light of their loss.

When and How to Make a Referral to Counseling

Often the most difficult parts of helping students is knowing when and how to refer them for further help. As higher education professionals, we have done our jobs well if we have developed strong relationships with our students and they feel safe and comfortable with us. But it is just as important for us to recognize when we can no longer give them the support they need—and refer them to counseling. Referrals can be tricky, however. While a student is grieving a loss, it is important that they not view this transfer to counseling as yet another loss of someone important.

Grieving is normal. Not every grieving student needs counseling. Higher education professionals should become concerned, however, when the grieving period begins to prolong suffering, interrupts normal activities, or prevents the student from living life to the fullest. Some students are unable to fully engage in the grieving process, which can lead to an unhealthy situation. Perhaps they cannot tolerate the pain associated with the loss, or they find the emotions that come with grieving simply too overwhelming. They may want to continue to interact with the deceased and cannot accept the fact that this person is truly gone. They might be feeling an overwhelming sense of guilt, either about the relationship with the person when they were alive or about their loved one's passing. For some, showing emotions such as crying is a sign of weakness. Perhaps they worry that by letting go of the pain, they are doing a disservice to the person they have lost.

Sometimes we do not know what to say to someone who is grieving. These responses, from the Josh Rojas Foundation (n.d), can be very useful:

> *"Feeling down, alone, sad, cranky, moody, tired, hopeless, angry, confused, and worse doesn't mean you are a failure. Your unhappiness is an expression of humanness."*
>
> *"Tears honor loss and relieve pent-up emotions."*
>
> *"Being depressed, quick to anger, weird in your humor, or wildly happy at odd times are all fairly common. As long as your behavior is not self-destructive or illegal, you're probably pretty normal."*
>
> *"If people can't be supportive, that's their problem. Find people who can understand."*
>
> *"You can carry your wound through life or help it to heal cleanly."*
>
> *"Having a tantrum will not hurry grief along. Your wound will heal naturally in its own time. Take great care of yourself in the meantime."*

When students are still not responding and seem unable to function due to grief, you should refer them to the counseling available on campus. The first step is knowing what's available. Some campuses offer support groups for grieving students. For many students, this option can be a good first step because they will be able to connect with peers going through something similar. Other students might prefer something more individual and personalized. In that case, a one-on-one counseling session might be better. Call ahead and explain to the counseling center professionals what the situation is with the student. They will offer some advice and perhaps even suggest a specific counselor. By calling ahead, you are already able to provide a lot of guidance and information to the student.

When making a referral to counseling, remember to let the student know why you are suggesting it. Point out the behaviors that concern you, using the empathy and techniques discussed in Chapter 2. Remind the student that they are not alone and offer to make the appointment with them. Let them know you will still be there to support them; referring them to counseling does not mean you are severing your ties. A referral is simply another way of letting a student know you care about them and their long-term success.

What Campuses Are Doing

Despite the need and calls in the literature for improved university support efforts (Balk, 2001), very few campuses have targeted interventions. In 2005, an organization called Actively Moving Forward (AMF) was created. AMF was founded *by* grieving college students *for* grieving college students. Unlike campus counseling centers, which serve the general population, AMF works with the specific population of students who are bereaved. It is a peer-led program, connecting grieving students with peers who understand what they are going through. AMF has reported that students find some comfort in helping others as well.

Programs like AMF have shown to be helpful. Another recommendation is to establish campus-based bereavement centers. These centers could focus on research, programs, and education. They could also provide the essential training needed not only for counselors but also for faculty, staff, and peers—perhaps even creating a peer grief counseling program. Peer counseling has proven effective in such areas as suicide prevention and other areas of mental health (Morse & Schulze, 2013).

Conclusion

Unfortunately, dealing with loss is a part of life. When bereavment occurs during the college years, it can be even more difficult. For many students, it may be their first time experiencing a loss, coupled with being away from home and without the support of their family. As they navigate through the stages of grief, students also have to figure out how to continue meeting academic and personal demands. They may feel that those around them do not really understand what they are going through, which might increase feelings of isolation and loneliness. When higher education professionals recognize the signs that a student is struggling, taking the time to talk with them and offer support and resources can be instrumental in helping the student move along the grieving process.

References

Balk, D. E. (2001). College student bereavement, scholarship, and the university: A call for university engagement. *Death Studies, 25*(1), 67–84. https://doi.org/10.1080/07481180126146

Balk, D. E. (2008). Grieving: 22–30% of all college students. In H. S. Servaty-Seib & D. J. Taub (Eds.), *Assisting bereaved college students* (pp. 5–14). Jossey-Bass

Balk, D. E., Tyson-Rawson, K., & Colletti-Wetzel, J. (1993). Social support as an intervention with bereaved college students. *Death Studies, 17*(5), 427–450. https://doi.org/10.1080/07481189308253387

Balk, D. E., & Vesta, L. C. (1998). Psychological development during 4 years of bereavement: A longitudinal case study. *Death Studies, 22*(1), 3–21. https://doi.org/10.1080/074811898201713

Bolden, L. A. (2007). A review of on grief and grieving: Finding the meaning of grief through the five stages of loss. *Counseling and Values, 51*(3), 235–237. https://doi.org/10.1002/j.2161-007X.2007.tb00081.x

Centers for Disease Control and Prevention. (2020). *Facts about suicide.* https://www.cdc.gov/suicide/facts/index.html

Cupit, I. N., Servaty-Seib, H. L., Parikh, S. T., A. Walker, A. C., & Martin, R. (2016). College and the grieving student: A mixed-methods analysis. *Death Studies, 40*(8), 494–506. https://doi.org/10.1080/07481187.2016.1181687

Fajgenbaum, D., Chesson, B., & Gaines Lanzi, R. (2012). Building a network of grief support on college campuses: A national grassroots initiative. *Journal of College Student Psychotherapy, 26*(2), 99–120.

Frazier, P., Anders, S., Perera, S., Tomich, P., Tennen, H., Park, C., & Tashiro, T. (2009). Traumatic events among undergraduate students: Prevalence and associated symptoms. *Journal of Consulting Psychology, 56*(3), 450–460. https://doi.org/10.1037/a0016412

Hardison, H. G., Neimeyer, R. A., & Lichstein, K. L. (2005). Insomnia and complicated grief symptoms in bereaved college students. *Behavioral Sleep Medicine, 3*(2), 99–111. https://doi.org/10.1207/s15402010bsm0302_4

HealGrief. (n.d.). *Understanding grief.* https://healgrief.org/understanding-grief

Josh Rojas Foundation. (n.d.). *7 healthy and unhealthy responses to grief.* http://www.joshrojas.org/responses.asp

King, A. R. (1998). Family environment scale predictors of academic performance. *Psychological Reports, 83,* 1319–1327.

Kübler-Ross, E. (1969). *On death and dying* (1st ed.). Routledge. https://doi.org/10.4324/9780203010495

Morse, C., & Schulze, R. (2013). Enhancing the network of peer support on college campuses. *Journal of College Student Psychotherapy, 27*(3), 212–225. https://doi.org/10.1080/87568225.2013.798222

National Action Alliance for Suicide Prevention and the Research Prioritization Task Force. (2014). *A prioritized research agenda for suicide prevention: An action plan to save lives.*

Oltjenbruns, K. A. (1996). Death of a friend during adolescence: Issues and impacts. In C. A. Corr & D. E. Balk (Eds.), *Handbook of adolescent death and bereavement* (pp. 196–215). Springer.

Servaty-Seib, H. L., & Hamilton, L. A. (2006). Educational performance and persistence of bereaved college students. *Journal of College Student Development, 47*(2), 225–234. https://doi.org/10.1353/csd.2006.0024

CHAPTER 14

Moving Forward

The goal of this book has been to give higher education professionals an introduction to the most common mental health issues they are likely to encounter in their daily work. The challenge is knowing just enough, but not so much that the knowledge becomes overwhelming. In a recent conversation with counseling center staff attending a Counseling Skills for Higher Education Professionals course taught by one of the authors of this book as part of a graduate higher education program, the staff members asked, "Are any of these students planning to become clinicians?" This was an important distinction, and a question that underscores why we wrote this book. Often, the classes offered to higher education professionals in their graduate preparation programs are part of a counseling program, not a higher education administration and student affairs program. Higher education students in these counseling classes often hear from the instructors of those courses, "This course isn't really for you" or "You don't really need to know this since you won't be doing counseling sessions." As a result, higher education professionals often are not given the training and preparation they need to respond when confronted with students having a mental health crisis.

As a higher education professional, you do not need to be an expert in mental health or counseling, but you do need a basic understanding of the etiologies of the issues students are facing. This book provides just that: a foundational knowledge of signs and symptoms, as well as guidance on how and when to intervene. You should have a clear understanding of the most common mental health concerns facing students and how the areas all fit together. The one common theme that ties college student mental health together is using the skill of empathy to support students in crisis. Think of a toolbox. Many tools can be used to tackle a project, but the one used the most often is the hammer. Empathy is the hammer: It is the tool that should be reached for first and most often. Then, other tools can be deployed once they are appropriate and needed. But it is the hammer, the *empathy*, that is the most important tool in the toolbox and is always needed the most.

Higher education professionals will be best served when they recognize they do not need to be experts in the areas of mental health covered in this book, but, rather, generalists who feel empowered to get involved when needed and to respond confidently when invited. Be confident in yourself and in your ability to listen and be empathetic. The hope is that after reading this book you will feel ready to reach out and connect with your students in meaningful ways. According to Cigna's (2018) U.S. Loneliness Index, Gen Z, or young people ages 18 to 22, are significantly more likely to be lonely than any other generation in the United States. Of those surveyed, 68% felt no one really knew them, 69% reported feeling shy, and 69% said they felt people around them were absent. Since this group is representative of traditional-aged college students, it is important to be aware of the sense of loneliness affecting this population. Understanding this generation's perspective on loneliness and belonging is a good starting place to make a difference. Higher education professionals, by nature of their close contact with students, are in unique positions to make a postive impact on these loneliness statistics by simply reaching out and talking with students about their daily lives and asking further questions when concerns arise. This book provides the knowledge and the skills needed to make these connections.

We shared the following statistics in Chapter 1, but they are worth repeating. Drum et al. (2009) found that among college students with serious suicidal ideation and attempts, 46% said they never talked to anyone else about these issues, and of those students who did talk to someone else, 67% of the time it was a peer, most often a close friend or roommate. Of those who talked about their struggles with others, only 52% found it helpful and only 58% were advised to seek professional help. This leaves many students with no real professional help for their often very serious, and potentially fatal, mental health issues. With the knowledge that has been gained from this book, you should feel empowered to step in and help students. You are now armed with increased information and an improved skill set. The hope is that these statistics can be improved and that more conversations between students in crisis and trusted faculty or staff members will be positive—perhaps resulting in a successful referral to a counseling center.

Sometimes the statistics can be overwhelming, and you might feel as though there is simply no way to do enough, help enough students, or make enough of an impact. There is a quote, mostly attributed to Maya Angelou circa 2014, that encapsulates much of what we aimed to accomplish in this book: "I have learned that people will forget what you did, people will forget what you said, but people will never forget how you made them feel." This is a good way to approach these conversations: Focus on feelings. Focus on listening. Focus on being present in the moment with each and every student and conversation. Focus on *empathy*.

We would like to end the book with a story that summarizes the overall message that what higher education professionals do matters. Every conversation can make a difference.

> ## The Starfish Story
>
> **Loren Eisely**
>
> One day a man was walking along the beach when he noticed a boy picking something up and gently throwing it into the ocean.
>
> Approaching the boy, he asked, "What are you doing?"
>
> The youth replied, "Throwing starfish back into the ocean. The surf is up and the tide is going out. If I don't throw them back, they'll die."
>
> "Son," the man said, "don't you realize there are miles and miles of beach and hundreds of starfish? You can't make a difference!"
>
> After listening politely, the boy bent down, picked up another starfish, and threw it back into the surf.
>
> Then, smiling at the man, he said, "I made a difference for that one."
>
> Make a difference for *that one*.

References

Cigna. (2018). *Cigna U.S. loneliness index*. https://www.multivu.com/players/English/8294451-cigna-us-loneliness-survey/docs/IndexReport_1524069371598-173525450.pdf

Drum, D. J., Brownson, C., Denmark, A. B., & Smith, S. E. (2009). New data on the nature of suicidal crises in college students: Shifting the paradigm. *Professional Psychology: Research and Practice, 40*(3), 213–222.

Appendix

Mental Health Resources

ANXIETY AND STRESS

Anxiety.org

https://www.anxiety.org/university-student-anxiety-resources

Anxiety.org is committed to making mental health information accessible, inclusive, easy to find, and simple to understand. Anxiety.org is an organization that wants anyone suffering from an anxiety disorder to have access to all the resources they need to understand and overcome their condition. The website contains the latest and most relevant information, by working directly with distinguished doctors, therapists, scientists, and specialists; it delivers to readers cutting-edge research and advancements in the field but keeps the content approachable. The goal of Anxiety.org is to bridge the understanding gap that exists between mental health professionals and those living with anxiety disorders.

Anxiety and Depression Association of America

https://adaa.org

The Anxiety and Depression Association of America (ADAA) is an international nonprofit membership organization dedicated to the prevention, treatment, and cure of anxiety, depression, obsessive compulsive disorder, posttraumatic stress disorder, and co-occurring disorders, through education, practice, and research. ADAA offers comprehensive services, including information on mental disorders by topic; free monthly webinars; podcasts; and access to treatment, community resources, informational videos, and blog posts.

Mental Health America

https://mhanational.org/conditions/anxiety

Mental Health America (MHA) is a national-level community-based nonprofit dedicated to addressing the needs of individuals living with mental illness. MHA works to promote mental health as a critical part of overall wellness, including prevention services for all; early identification and intervention for those at risk; integrated care, services, and supports for those who need them, with recovery as the goal. MHA's programs and initiatives promote mental health and aid with the prevention of mental illness, through advocacy, education, research, and services. MHA has more than 200 affiliate offices around the United States that work every day to protect the rights and dignity of individuals with lived experience and ensure that peers and their voices are integrated into all areas of the organization.

National Alliance on Mental Illness

https://nami.org/About-Mental-Illness/Mental-Health-Conditions/Anxiety-Disorders

The National Alliance on Mental Illness (NAMI) is a grassroots mental health organization dedicated to building better lives for millions of Americans affected by mental illness. Its focus is on helping raise awareness and providing support and education for those in need. NAMI offers advocacy, education, support, and public awareness so that individuals and families affected by mental illness. The core values of NAMI include hope, inclusion, empowerment, compassion, and fairness. NAMI provides work equity and inclusion to anyone suffering from mental illness regardless of gender, race, gender identity, ethnicity, national origin, age, sexual orientation, education, disability, veteran status, or other dimension of diversity.

National Institute of Mental Health: Anxiety Disorders

https://www.nimh.nih.gov/health/education-awareness/shareable-resources-on-anxiety-disorders.shtml

The National Institute of Mental Health (NIMH) is the lead federal agency for research on mental health disorders. Its mission is to transform the understanding and treatment of mental illnesses through research, to pave the way for prevention, recovery, and cure. NIMH has resources catered to different mental health topics. Its webpage on anxiety disorders offers shareable graphics, brochures, fact sheets, social media messages, videos, and statistics. Its information resource center features a hotline and online chatting services available to those seeking additional information.

BOUNDARIES AND CONFIDENTIALITY

Clery Center

https://clerycenter.org

The Clery Center is a national nonprofit dedicated to helping college and university officials meet the standards of the Clery Act.

DEPRESSION AND SUICIDE

Active Minds

https://www.activeminds.org

Many schools have student-run chapters of Active Minds on their campuses. Active Minds was founded by Alison Malmon when she was a junior at the University of Pennsylvania after she lost her older brother to suicide. Active Minds focuses on helping student raise awareness about mental health and suicide by opening dialogue and reducing stigma

American Foundation for Suicide Prevention

https://afsp.org

This website provides links to a multitude of suicide prevention resources.

The Jed Foundation

https://jedfoundation.org

The Jed Foundation is a nonprofit that protects emotional health and prevents suicide for teens and young adults. It partners with high schools and colleges to strengthen their mental health, substance misuse, and suicide prevention programs and systems. It focuses on equipping teens and young adults with the skills and knowledge they need to help themselves and each other. It encourages community awareness, understanding, and action for young adult mental health.

National Suicide Prevention Lifeline

1-800-273-TALK (8255)

This resource provides 24-7 free and confidential support for people in distress, prevention and crisis resources, and best practices for professionals.

Question, Persuade, Refer

https://qprinstitute.com

Question, Persuade, Refer (QPR) is a three-step suicide prevention training program that teaches individuals how to recognize the warning signs of suicide and how to **q**uestion, **p**ersuade, and **r**efer a person in crisis. Anyone can become QPR trained and certified, but many campuses have chosen to implement this training for faculty and staff.

Suicide Prevention Resource Center

https://sprc.org

The Suicide Prevention Resource Center is the only federally supported resource center devoted to advancing the implementation of the National Strategy for Suicide Prevention, which is funded by SAMHSA.

Student Support Network

With the support of a SAMHSA grant, the Student Development and Counseling Center at Worcester Polytechnic Institute (WPI), a midsize university in the Northeast, developed and implemented a broad-based, student-centered training program intended to improve the network of peer support on campus. The program identified and trained a range of connected and concerned students in how to recognize and support other students in distress and when and how to connect their peers with professional help for mental health concerns. Once trained, these students become part of the university's Student Support Network, a group dedicated to and supported in reaching out and helping other students in distress. WPI made this program available to campuses across the country, and many have implemented it to help with suicide prevention.

EATING DISORDERS

Academy for Eating Disorders

https://www.aedweb.org

The Academy for Eating Disorders (AED) is a global professional association committed to leadership in eating disorders research, education, treatment, and prevention. The goal of AED is to provide global access to knowledge, research, and best treatment practices for eating disorders. AED helps physicians, psychiatrists, psychologists, nutritionists, academic researchers, students, and those with lived experience connect and collaborate with each other and keep abreast of recent developments in eating disorders research. The website also offers a range of resources, including fast facts on eating disorders, treatment options, access to publications and continuing education credits, webinars, and additional resources for professionals, students, and those who have experience with eating disorders.

Eating Disorders Coalition

http://www.eatingdisorderscoalition.org

The Eating Disorders Coalition is a federal advocacy organization for eating disorders. Its mission is to advance the federal recognition of eating disorders as a public health priority, working with Congress to effectively influence policy. The website offers facts and information on a variety of topics concerning eating disorders. The user can access information sheets or be redirected to websites that operate hotlines and other services useful for those suffering from eating disorders and for their support systems. The Eating Disorders Coalition encourages users to visit its member organizations for more facts and information. It also offers a link to the Eating Disorders Information Gateway. By requesting a free account, the user will have access to a plethora of useful information regarding eating disorders and recovery.

National Alliance for Eating Disorders

https://www.allianceforeatingdisorders.com

The National Alliance for Eating Disorders is a national nonprofit organization dedicated to providing programs and activities aimed at outreach, education, early intervention, and advocacy for all eating disorders. The alliance offers comprehensive services, including educational presentations to schools, health care providers, hospitals, treatment centers, and community agencies; free, clinician-led weekly support groups for those struggling and for their loved ones; support and referrals through both its free helpline and comprehensive referral website, www.findEDhelp.com; and advocacy for eating disorders and mental health legislation.

National Eating Disorders Association

https://www.nationaleatingdisorders.org

The National Eating Disorders Association (NEDA) is the largest nonprofit organization dedicated to supporting individuals and families affected by eating disorders. It has taken on major roles in advocacy, research, educational content, support for individuals and families, local engagement, and national partnerships. The website provides access to screening tools, treatment providers, low-cost support options, and information on recovery and relapse. NEDA also operates a confidential hotline for help. This site also includes a list of colleges and what support they offer.

GRIEF AND LOSS

Coalition to Support Grieving Students

https://grievingstudents.org

This website contains useful information for parents and students. It features modules with helpful material as well as articles and pamphlets with tips and advice.

Eluna

https://elunanetwork.org/national-bereavement-resource-guide/resources

Eluna is a public, 501(c)(3) nonprofit organization with a mission to provide comfort, hope, and healing to children affected by loss and family addiction. The organization offers a guide with a compilation of state and local resources—camps and grief organizations organized by state, plus books and websites for children and their families experiencing loss. Although this site is primarily for children, there are a number of resources useful for people of all ages.

INTERPERSONAL VIOLENCE

Esperanza United

https://esperanzaunited.org/en

Esperanza United is a leader in the domestic violence movement and a national resource center for organizations working with Latinas in the United States. Based in St. Paul, Minnesota, Casa de Esperanza's mission is to "mobilize Latinas and Latinx communities to end domestic violence." Founded in 1982 to provide emergency shelter for Latinas and other women and children experiencing domestic violence, the organization has grown to become the largest Latina organization in the country focused on domestic violence. Esperanza United is also committed to becoming a greater resource to organizations and communities in the areas of sexual assault and trafficking. Esperanza United's leadership in the field has been recognized by the U.S. Department of Health and Human Services, which has designated the organization as the Culturally Specific Issue Resource Center on Domestic Violence and Latinx Communities. What makes Esperanza United so beneficial for students is that it provides bilingual services and also bilingual resources in both Spanish and English.

LoveIsRespect

https://www.loveisrespect.org

LoveisRespect is a national resource to disrupt and prevent unhealthy relationships and IPV by empowering young people through inclusive and equitable education, support, and resources. Originally developed by the National Domestic Violence Hotline, this project aims to give information, support, and advocacy to young people ages 13 to 26 who may have questions or concerns about romantic relationships. This national resource also provides support for concerned friends, family members, teachers, counselors, and other service providers through free and confidential services via phone, text, and live chat. In addition, this resource has comprehensive education, including quizzes, interactive pages, and testimonials, as well as training, toolkits, and curriculum for educators, peers, and parents to promote healthy relationships and prevent future abuse.

National Center for Victims of Crime: Stalking Resource Center

https://victimsofcrime.org/stalking-resource-center

The National Center for Victims of Crime and the U.S. Department of Justice Office on Violence Against Women partnered to create the Stalking Resource Center (SRC). It promotes awareness, action, and advocacy to enhance victim safety and hold offenders of stalking accountable. SRC's mission is to enhance the ability of professionals, organizations, and systems to respond to stalking effectively. The website offers information about federal, tribal, state, and military stalking statutes, a guide to online resources, practitioner profiles, a national helpline for victims, and more.

National Center on Domestic Violence, Trauma & Mental Health

http://www.nationalcenterdvtraumamh.org

The National Center on Domestic Violence, Trauma & Mental Health provides training, support, and consultation to advocates, mental health and substance abuse providers, legal professionals, and policymakers as they work to improve agency- and systems-level responses to survivors and their children. The work of the center is to give survivors defined support rooted in principles of social justice. This center is one of four Special Issue Resource Centers funded by the U.S. Department of Health and Human Services working under the Domestic Violence Resource Center.

National Coalition Against Domestic Violence

https://ncadv.org/resources

The National Coalition Against Domestic Violence (NCADV) seeks to lead, mobilize, and raise voices to support efforts that demand a change of those conditions that lead to domestic violence, such as patriarchy, privilege, racism, sexism, and classism. NCADV is dedicated to supporting survivors and advocates and holding offenders accountable. Some of the resources address education and sharing information about sexual abuse and domestic violence.

NCADV builds support networks through membership and gives financial education and support for those individuals in situations that require it.

National Domestic Violence Hotline

https://www.thehotline.org

The National Domestic Violence Hotline has essential tools and support to help survivors of domestic violence live their lives free of abuse. The hotline provides high-trained expert advocates for free. The service provided is kept confidential. The individuals working with the hotline are compassionate, supportive, and deliver crisis information, education, and referral sources in 200 different languages. The goal for the National Domestic Violence Hotline is to free all victims of violent relationships and provide them with support to allow survivors to shift the power back onto themselves. The hotline's approach focuses on integrity, thought leadership, excellence, collaboration, social justice, and caring, and it is survivor oriented.

The Red Flag Campaign

http://www.theredflagcampaign.org

Available for purchase by colleges and universities, the Red Flag Campaign can be used as a public awareness campaign on campus. It employs a bystander intervention strategy to address and prevent sexual assault, dating violence, and stalking on college campuses. The campaign encourages friends and other campus community members to say something when they see warning signs ("red flags") for sexual assault, dating violence, or stalking in a friend's relationship.

SEXUAL ASSAULT AND VICTIMIZATION

Futures Without Violence

https://www.futureswithoutviolence.org/campus

Futures Without Violence is a nonprofit organization that works to end a number of gender-based violence issues, including sexual assault and domestic violence. Its website offers educational resources for providers, staff, and student health educators on college campuses.

National Center for Victims of Crime

https://victimsofcrime.org

The National Center for Victims of Crime is a nonprofit organization that advocates for victims' rights, trains professionals who work with victims, and provides information on victims' issues. The National Center for Victims of Crime is one of the most comprehensive national resources committed to advancing victims' rights and helping victims of crime rebuild their lives. The National Center addresses all types of crime, including victims of sexual assault. It provides direct services to site visitors, such as attorney referrals, confidential help lines, and interactive trainings.

National Center on Domestic and Sexual Violence

http://www.ncdsv.org/ncd_about.html

The National Center on Domestic and Sexual Violence helps professionals who work with victims and perpetrators; law enforcement; criminal justice professionals, such as prosecutors, judges, and probation officers; health care professionals, including emergency response teams, nurses, and doctors; domestic violence and sexual assault advocates and service providers; and counselors and social workers.

The website includes links to publications, training opportunities, and relevant news.

National Sexual Violence Resource Center

https://www.nsvrc.org

The National Sexual Violence Resource Center (NSVRC) is the leading nonprofit in providing information and tools to prevent and respond to sexual violence. This center provides resources and education to help survivors of sexual assault. NSVRC translates research and trends into best practices that help individuals, communities, and service providers achieve real and lasting change. NSVRC also works with the media to promote informed reporting. Every April, NSVRC leads Sexual Assault Awareness Month, a campaign to educate and engage the public in addressing this widespread issue.

Rape, Abuse & Incest National Network

https://www.rainn.org

The Rape, Abuse & Incest National Network (RAINN) is the nation's largest anti-sexual violence organization and leading authority on sexual violence. The organization is comprised of experts in victim services, public education, public policy, consulting services, and technology that provides best-in-class services for survivors, informs and educates the nation about sexual violence, and improves the public policy and criminal justice response to sexual violence. RAINN created and operates the National Sexual Assault Hotline, accessible 24-7 by phone (800.656.HOPE) and online (https://hotline.rainn.org/online). The organization works closely with many local sexual assault service providers to offer confidential support services to survivors regardless of where they are in their recovery. The website also offers warning signs for students and loved ones and toolkits for organizations to use that help people connect with RAINN services.

SUBSTANCE ABUSE

Alcoholics Anonymous

https://aa.org

Alcoholics Anonymous (AA) is an international fellowship of men and women who have had a drinking problem. It is nonprofessional, self-supporting, multiracial, apolitical, and available almost everywhere. There are no age or education requirements. Membership is open to anyone who wants to do something about their drinking problem. There is an app that can help people find support meetings. AA is an international mutual aid fellowship with the stated purpose of enabling its members to "stay sober and help other alcoholics achieve sobriety." Its concept revolves around the premise that alcoholism is an illness that can be managed but not controlled. AA's 12-step approach follows a set of guidelines designed as "steps" toward recovery, and members can revisit these steps at any time. Since the meetings are easily accessible and free to attend, AA is recognized as an important aid to recovery.

Faces and Voices of Recovery

https://facesandvoicesofrecovery.org/resources

Faces and Voice of Recovery is an organization with a mission to support individuals in long-term recovery from drug and alcohol addictions. It also supports family, friends, and allies through capacity building in support of the national recovery movement, fighting the stigma of addiction, and creating recovery messaging trainings. The website provides access to resources for COVID-19, webinars, publications, and a resource library. The organization advocates for recovery support services nationwide and provides guidance and expertise on implementing effective recovery support services. Another notable service the organization offers is a guide to mutual aid resources available to individuals wishing to participate in long-term recovery as well as to their family or loved ones.

National Institute on Alcohol Abuse and Alcoholism

https://www.niaaa.nih.gov/about-niaaa

The National Institute on Alcohol Abuse and Alcoholism (NIAAA) is one of the 27 institutes and centers that comprise the National Institutes of Health. NIAAA supports and conducts research on the impact of alcohol use on human health and well-being. It is the largest funder of alcohol research in the world. The mission of NIAAA is to generate and disseminate fundamental knowledge about the effects of alcohol on health and well-being and to apply that knowledge to improve diagnosis, prevention, and treatment of alcohol-related problems, including alcohol use disorder, across the life span. The website contains pages devoted to the problem of college drinking, including fact sheets and links to other resources.

National Institute on Drug Abuse

https://www.drugabuse.gov

The mission of the National Institute on Drug Abuse (NIDA) is to advance science on the causes and consequences of drug use and addiction and to apply that knowledge to improve individual and public health. NIDA supports and conducts basic and clinical research on drug use (including nicotine), its consequences, and the underlying neurobiological, behavioral, and social mechanisms involved. Another goal is to ensure the effective translation, implementation, and dissemination of scientific research findings to improve the prevention and treatment of substance use disorders and enhance public awareness of addiction as a brain disorder. NIDA's website provides screening tools, prevention efforts, and treatment resources for those suffering from substance abuse disorders.

Substance Abuse and Mental Health Services Administration

https://www.samhsa.gov/families

The Substance Abuse and Mental Health Services Administration (SAMHSA) was established by the U.S. Congress and is the agency within the U.S. Department of Health and Human Services that leads public health efforts to advance behavioral health. SAMHSA's mission is to reduce the impact of mental health and substance abuse on America's communities. Its website offers resources for families coping with mental health and substance abuse disorders; emphasizes the role of support in the healing process; and provides videos, guides, relevant references, and links to access help, as well as the national help hotline.

The Authors

Maureen C. Kenny is a licensed psychologist at Florida International University. She is a member of the Applied Social and Cultural Psychology Program and has over 25 years' experience in academia teaching graduate counseling courses with a diverse student body. Kenny is a member of the American Counseling Association and a Fellow of the American Psychological Association. She is the past recipient of a number of awards from the Florida Psychological Association, including Outstanding Member Award (2000, 2014), What A Woman Award (2009), Creative Marketing Award (2000), and Early Career Contributions to Psychology (1997). She is also the recipient of the 2000 Distinguished Alumni Achievement Award from the Center for Psychological Studies at Nova Southeastern University. In 2019, she was the inaugural recipient of the Citizen Psychologist Award from Division 37 of the American Psychological Association. In 2021, she received the Locke Paisley Outstanding Mentor Award from the Association of Counselor Education and Supervision.

Kenny is the author of over 75 journal articles and serves on the editorial board of a number of journals, including *Journal of Child Sexual Abuse, Journal of Child and Adolescent Trauma,* and *Psychological Trauma: Theory, Research and Practice.* She is the editor of *Sex Education: Attitude of Adolescents, Cultural Differences and Schools' Challenges* (Nova Science Publishers, 2015) and co-author with Jan Moursand of *The Process of Counseling and Therapy* (Prentice Hall, 2002).

As a clinician, Kenny has worked in south Florida as a licensed psychologist with abused children and adult survivors of trauma. Trained in trauma-focused cognitive behavioral therapy, she uses a trauma-informed approach to working with clients.

Kenny earned a BA in psychology at Rutgers College, and an MS and PhD in clinical psychology from Nova Southeastern University. She completed a doctoral internship at Children's Psychiatric Center in Miami, Florida. Her postdoctoral fellowship was at the Child and Adolescent Traumatic Stress Program at Nova Southeastern University.

Rebekah F. Schulze is a clinical associate professor of higher education at Florida International University. Schulze joined the Florida International University community in 2014 as the founding director of scholar development. She has been a member of the faculty since 2015 and has served as the graduate program director as well as an Honors College Fellow.

Schulze has worked at several higher education institutions in a variety of roles, including associate dean of students, assistant dean for academic support services, director of residence life and judicial affairs, and director of orientation. She worked in the counseling center at Worcester Polytechnic Institute of Technology, where she was involved with peer education and suicide prevention efforts.

Schulze earned a BA from Colby College; an MA in administration, leadership, and technology from New York University; and an EdD in educational leadership and development from Boston University. Her research area is mental health for college students and counseling skills for higher education professionals. She publishes articles, presents, and teaches classes in this field.

Index

Figures and tables are indicated by "f" and "t" following the page numbers.

A

Abusive relationships. *See* Interpersonal violence
Academic issues
    anxiety and, 72, 78, 81–82, 84
    depression and, 93
    grief and, 186–188
    interpersonal violence and, 150
    LGBTQIA+ students and, 64
    stress and, 76
    substance use and, 168–169, 170
Accommodations, 64, 84
Acculturation, 60
ACHA. *See* American College Health Association
ACPA–College Student Educators International, 17–18, 51, 52
Acquaintance rape, 127–128, 134–135
Actively Moving Forward (AMF), 190
Activism, 68
Acute stress, 45, 76
Adaptability, 49–50, 76, 81
Adderall, 162, 168–169
Addictions counseling, 174–175
ADHD (attention deficit hyperactivity disorder), 168
Advice and problem solving, 8, 20–21, 37, 115
Affirming, 36
Alcoholics Anonymous, 175
Alcohol use, 160, 163, 164–166, 170. *See also* Substance use and abuse
Alley, Z. M., 166–167
American College Health Association (ACHA)
    on anxiety, 72, 74
    on eating disorders, 105
    on interpersonal violence, 145
    on stalking, 149
    on stress, 75–76
    on substance use, 160, 168
    on suicide and depression, 1–2, 87, 92
American Council on Education, 1
American Psychiatric Association (APA), 89, 110
Americans with Disabilities Act (1990), 64
AMF (Actively Moving Forward), 190
Angelou, Maya, 195
Annual security reports (ASRs), 31
Anorexia nervosa, 109–110
Anticipatory stress, 76
Anxiety. *See also* Stress
    activities to reduce, 81–82
    approaching students with, 78–82
    backpack metaphor for, 3–4
    case studies on, 72–74, 79
    counseling referrals for, 82–84
    depression and, 82, 90
    resources for, 197–199
    sexual assault and, 128–129
    statistics on, 2, 72, 74
    symptoms of, 71–75
    test anxiety, 78

APA (American Psychiatric Association), 89, 110
Approaching students
    with anxiety, 78–82
    with depression or suicidal ideation, 96–98
    with eating disorders, 112–116
    with grief, 185–188
    on interpersonal violence issues, 150–155, 154*t*
    on sexual assault and victimization experiences, 130–135, 134*t*
    on substance use, 171–173
ASRs (annual security reports), 31
Associated Press poll, 95
Association of American Universities, 145
Athletics, 106, 162–163
Attending behaviors, 10–12
Attention deficit hyperactivity disorder (ADHD), 168
Attrition rates, 47
Autism spectrum, 65

B

Backpack metaphor, 3–4
Bamber, M. D., 75, 80, 81
Barkhuizen, N., 48
Benson, K., 168
Bereavement. *See* Grief and loss
Bias, 17–18, 67
Binge drinking, 163, 165, 170
Binge eating and purging, 76, 109–110, 112
Biofeedback, 83
BIPOC (Black, Indigenous, and People of Color) students, 61–63
Bipolar disorder, 92

Black Lives Matter movement, 60–61
Blaming victims, 131–132, 134
Body dysmorphia, 114
Body image. *See* Eating disorders
Body language, 10–11
Borders, L. D., 166
Borshuk, C., 26
Boundaries and confidentiality, 25–32
    FERPA and, 28–30
    mandatory reporting under Clery Act, 30–31
    overview, 26–27
    privacy of student and, 37–38
    relationship development and, 27–28
    resources for, 199
Breathing exercises, 81
Buckley, James, 28
Buckman, J. F., 163
Bulimia nervosa, 110–112
Bullying, 68–69
Burke, M. G., 171
Burnout, 46–49
Byrd-Bredbenner, C., 108

C

CAGE screening method for alcohol use, 173
Campus crime statistics, 30–31
Career indecision, 75
Carmody, D., 149
Case studies
    on anxiety and stress, 72–74, 79
    on depression and suicide, 89, 94
    on eating disorders, 104, 106–107, 111
    on grief, 183
    on interpersonal violence, 144, 147

on sexual assault and
victimization, 126–128
on substance abuse, 162, 165
Cass, A. I., 150
Casual sex, 125
Catastrophizing, 77
CBT (cognitive-behavioral
therapy), 83
Center for Collegiate Mental
Health, 118
Centers for Disease Control and
Prevention (CDC), 94
Change and change model
action stage, 35
contemplation stage, 34–35
magic number theory and, 38
maintenance stage, 35–36
motivational interviewing
and, 36–37
precontemplation stage, 34
preparation stage, 35
Prochaska's stages, 34–36
reaching out, considerations
for, 37–38
Changing the subject, 13
CHOICE community, 161
Chronic stress, 45–46
Cigna U.S. Loneliness Index, 194
Clery Disclosure of Campus Security
Policy and Campus Crime Statistics
Act (1990), 30–31
Closed-ended questions, 13
Clubs and organizations,
65–66, 68, 190. *See also* Greek-
letter organizations
Cognitive-behavioral therapy
(CBT), 83
Cognitive reappraisal, 80
College Parents of America, 76

Competency areas for student affairs
educators, 17–18, 51, 52
Concentration and focus
depression and, 90
eating disorders and, 116
grief and, 186
self-care and, 52
sexual assault victims and, 129
stress and, 76, 77
substance use and, 168
Confidence, 49–50
Confidentiality. *See* Boundaries
and confidentiality
Confrontation, 19–20, 174. *See also*
Approaching students
Connection wellness, 52
Cooper, C. L., 49
Coping skills
burnout and, 48
crises vs., 39
eating disorders and, 114
homesickness and, 77
maladaptive, 45, 81
self-advocacy and, 68
stress and, 45–46, 80
substance use and, 166, 172
for triggers, 19
Corey, G., 46–47, 51, 52
Coulter, R. W. S., 125
Counseling, defined, 7–8
Counseling centers and services
client per counselor case loads
for, 118
confidentiality and, 28
cultural attitudes on, 39
cultural representation in
hiring, 66
grief and, 185
referrals to. *See* Referrals to
counseling centers

statistics on, 2
student awareness of, 98
student groups formed by, 68
suicide and, 95–96, 98–99
Counseling skills, 7–23
   advice and problem solving, 19–20
   attending, 10–12
   confrontation and, 19–20
   higher education and, 7–8
   listening, 9–10
   neutral manner of responding, 17
   paraphrasing, 15–17
   questions, use of, 12–13
   rapport, 9
   reflecting feeling, 14
   summarizing, 14–15
   triggers, management of, 18–19
   values, challenges to, 17–18
Crime, 30–31. *See also* Interpersonal violence; Sexual assault and victimization
Crises. *See also* Suicide and suicidal ideation
   advice giving and, 21
   help-seeking behaviors for, 2, 98
   referrals to counseling centers and, 39
Cultural and diversity awareness, 59–70
   attending and, 10–11
   BIPOC students, 61–63
   counseling, attitudes toward, 39
   current climate and, 60–61
   demographic changes and, 59–60
   eating disorders and, 108
   higher education enrollment statistics and, 59–60, 60*t*
   LGBTQIA+ students, 63–64
   on-campus support for, 66
   questions, awareness in asking, 13
   sexual assault and victimization, 131
   students with disabilities, 64–66
   suicide risk and, 92–93
   training and professional development on, 67–68
Culture of college, 160
Cupit, I. N., 187
Cyberstalking, 149

D

Dating relationships, 77. *See also* Interpersonal violence
Davis, R. E., 169, 170
Deaths, 110. *See also* Grief and loss; Suicide and suicidal ideation
Demographic changes, 59–60
Denial of problems, 113
Department of Education (DOE, U.S.), 29, 30–31
Depressants. *See* Substance use and abuse
Depression. *See also* Suicide and suicidal ideation
   anxiety and, 82, 90
   approaching students and, 96–98
   bipolar disorder and, 92
   burnout and, 48
   case studies on, 89, 94
   help-seeking behavior for, 98
   overview, 87
   resilience and, 51
   resources for, 199–201
   sexual assault and, 128
   signs and symptoms of, 88–91, 90*t*, 91*f*
   stage of grief, 184
   student work–life balance and, 75

Diagnostic and Statistical Manual of Mental Disorders, Fifth Edition (DSM-5)
    on depression, 89–90
    on eating disorders, 105, 108–109, 110
    on substance abuse disorders, 170–171
Dieting. *See* Eating disorders
Disabilities, students with, 64–66, 84, 168
Disability resource offices, 84
Discrimination. *See* Cultural and diversity awareness
Domestic violence. *See* Interpersonal violence
Druckman, J. N., 163
Drug use. *See* Substance use and abuse
Drum, D. J., 2, 98, 195

E

Eating disorders, 103–121
    approaching students with, 112–116
    case studies on, 104, 106–107, 111
    referrals to counseling for, 116–118
    resources for, 202–203
    signs and symptoms of, 103–108
    suicide and, 110, 118
    types of, 108–112
Educational records, 29–30
Edwards, K. M., 148
Eisely, Loren, 196
Embarrassment, 74, 115
Emotional abuse. *See* Interpersonal violence
Emotions. *See also* Grief and loss; *specific emotions*
    conveying through comments and behavior, 10
    depression and, 88–91, 90*t*
    reflecting feeling and, 14
    sexual assault disclosure and, 132–133
    triggers and, 18–19, 94, 106, 173
Empathy
    attending skills and, 10
    counseling skills and, 8
    eating disorders and, 115
    emotional wellness and, 52
    grief and, 185
    motivational interviewing and, 36
    reaching out, 38
    sexual assault disclosures and, 131
    substance use disorders and, 172, 174
    suicidality and, 96
    as tool, 5, 194
    training and professional development, 67
Employment of students, 75
Empowerment, 8, 21
Encouragers, 11–12
Ending meetings, 15
Ethics and confidentiality, 25
Ethnicity. *See* Cultural and diversity awareness
Eustis, E. H., 81–82
Exercise, 52, 105, 111
Exhaustion, 46–49
Eye contact, 9, 10–11

F

Faculty and staff. *See also* Self-care
    boundaries and confidentiality, 26–27
    cultural representation in hiring, 66
    in loco parentis and, 26

student mental health issues
and, 4–5
training on cultural
awareness, 67–68
training on mental health
crises, 193–194
Family Educational Rights and
Privacy Act (FERPA, 1974),
25, 28–30
Family-of-origin violence, 148
Family Policy Compliance Office of
DOE, 29
Fatigue, 46–49
Fear, 73–74, 84, 109, 149–150. *See
also* Anxiety
Financial issues, 75
Focus. *See* Concentration and focus
Ford, J., 125
Franko, D. L., 105
Fraternities. *See* Greek-
letter organizations
Frazier, P., 182
Freudenberger, Herbert, 46
Friendships, 77, 98, 129, 186

G

Garrett Lee Smith Memorial Act
(2004), 99
Gender. *See also* Sexual assault
and victimization
eating disorders and, 105–107,
109, 110–111, 113, 116
interpersonal violence and, 148
substance use and, 163–164,
166, 168–169
suicide risk and, 92–93
Generalized anxiety disorder, 73
Generation Z, 194–195
Genuineness, 8

Goals
motivational interviewing and, 36
test anxiety and, 78
wellness and, 52
Gonzaga University v. Doe (2002), 29
Good faith reporting of criminal
allegations, 30–31
Grades. *See* Academic issues
Greek-letter organizations, 17,
106–107, 162, 163–164
Grief and loss, 181–192
acceptance stage, 184
anger stage, 184
approaching students with, 185–188
bargaining stage, 184
campus-based resources for, 190
case study on, 183
counseling referrals for, 188–190
denial stage, 184
depression stage, 184
resources for, 204
signs and symptoms of, 181–185
Grossbard, J. R., 165

H

Hagedorn, L. S., 77
Hakanen, J. J., 48
Hallucinogens. *See* Substance use
and abuse
Harassment, 68–69, 149–150
Hardy, A., 130
Haven Sober Living Residences, 175
Health Insurance Portability and
Accountability Act (HIPAA,
1996), 25
The Healthy Minds Network, 88, 95
Hearing-impaired students, 65
Hettler, Bill, 52

Higher education professionals. *See* Faculty and staff
Hobbies, 53, 81
Homesickness, 10, 77
Homework, 78, 80–81
Hopelessness, 89
The Hunting Ground (documentary), 124

I

"I" statements, 114
Identity development, 125–126, 161
Illness, 45
Immune system and health, 76
Imposter syndrome, 61–62
Inclusive language, 65
Information giving, 20–21, 40
Inhalants. *See* Substance use and abuse
In loco parentis, 26
Insomnia, 82, 186
Interpersonal violence (IPV), 143–158
    approaching students on, 150–155, 154*t*
    case studies on, 144, 147
    overview, 143
    referrals to counseling centers for, 155–156
    resources for, 204–207
    signs and symptoms of, 144–149, 146*t*
    stalking and, 149–150
Isolation and loneliness
    eating disorders and, 116, 128
    Generation Z and, 194–195
    grief and, 185–186
    interpersonal violence and, 145
    substance use and, 169
    suicide and depression, 96

IS PATH WARM mnemonic for suicide risk, 91, 91*f*
"It's On Us" campaign (2014), 124
Ivey, Alan, 7, 11, 13

J

Jealousy, 146
Johnson, S. J., 51
Josh Rojas Foundation, 189

K

Kaukinen, C., 146, 147
Kraenzle Schneider, J., 75, 81
Krebs, C. P., 127
Kübler-Ross, E., 183

L

Lambert, E. G., 149–150
Law enforcement
    sexual victimization and, 131
    stalking and, 150, 156
Learning disabilities, 84, 168
Lehigh University CHOICE community, 161
Leiter, M. P., 47–48
Lewis, J. A., 173
LGBTQIA+ students
    cultural diversity and awareness, 63–64
    eating disorders and, 107–108, 112
    interpersonal violence and, 148
    sexual victimization and, 125, 131
    substance use and, 162, 164, 175
    suicide risk and, 92–93
Likis-Werle, E., 166, 173
Lipson, S. K., 108

Listening, 8, 9–10, 97. *See also* Approaching students
Loneliness. *See* Isolation and loneliness
Loss. *See* Grief and loss

M

Magic number theory, 38
Mahmoud, J. S. R., 81
Mandatory reporting, 30–31
Manning, P., 164
Marijuana use, 160, 167–168, 167t, 170. *See also* Substance use and abuse
Maslach, C., 47–48
Mason, B., 146
McCabe, S. E., 163–164
Medications
    for anxiety, 83–84
    misuse of, 160, 168–169
Meditation, 81
Meetings, 15
Men. *See* Gender
Mental health issues. *See also* Anxiety; Depression; Suicide and suicidal ideation
    campus-based responses to, 98–100
    race and ethnicity, 62
    statistics on, 1–2
    stigma and, 3, 62–63
    stress and, 46
    substance use and, 162
Mental health resources, 197–212
#MeToo movement, 124
Mindfulness-based interventions, 80, 81
Mind wellness, 52
Minority status stress, 62

Mobility issues, 65
Mood disorders, 92
Morpeth, E., 80
Morse, Charlie, 3–4
Motivational interviewing (MI), 36–37
mtvU poll, 95

N

NASPA–Student Affairs Administrators in Higher Education, 17–18, 51, 52
National Center for Education Statistics, 59
National College Health Assessment (ACHA), 1, 72, 74, 75–76, 98
National Collegiate Athletic Association (NCAA), 163
National Eating Disorders Collaboration, 114
National Institute on Drug Abuse, 161
Natrajan-Tyagi, R., 9
Nonjudgment
    counseling response and, 17, 18
    eating disorders and, 115
    interpersonal violence and, 152
    listening and, 10
    mindfulness and, 81
    sexual assault victims and, 134, 137
    substance use and, 173
    suicidality and, 96
Nonverbal language, 10–11, 20, 65

O

Obama, Barack, 124
Ohrt, J. H., 52, 54
Open-ended questions, 13, 36

Opioids, 167t, 169. *See also* Substance use and abuse

P

Panic attacks, 74, 82, 83–84
Paraphrasing, 15–17
Parents
    educational record access and, 29–30
    expectations as source of student stress, 76
    interpersonal violence and, 148
    new independence from, 72, 114, 160
Parks, A. C., 46
Parties and social events, 160
Peer pressure, 161
Pelletier, J. E., 80
Perfectionism, 116
Performance-enhancing drugs, 163, 168–169
Personal information. *See* Boundaries and confidentiality
Person-first language, 65
Phobias, 73, 84
Physical abuse. *See* Interpersonal violence; Sexual assault and victimization
Physical health
    anxiety and, 73
    body wellness and, 52, 53
    burnout and, 47–48
    depression and, 90
    eating disorders. *See* Eating disorders
    grief and, 186
    sleep issues and, 82, 90, 92, 186
    stress and, 45–46, 76

Posttraumatic stress disorder (PTSD), 128–130, 135, 166
Pregnancy, 136–137
Prescription medications. *See* Substance use and abuse
Privacy. *See* Boundaries and confidentiality
Problem solving and advice, 8, 20–21, 37, 115
Prochaska's stages of change model, 34–36
Professional Competency Areas for Student Affairs Educators (ACPA & NASPA), 17–18, 51, 52
Professional development, 67–68, 193–194
Pryce, J. G., 48
Psychological resources, 76–77
Psychosomatic symptoms, 73
PTSD (posttraumatic stress disorder), 128–130, 135, 166
Purposefulness, 50, 53

Q

Questioning techniques, 12–13, 36, 154, 172
Quick, V. M., 108

R

Race. *See* Cultural and diversity awareness
Racism, 62, 63, 68
Rape. *See* Sexual assault and victimization
Rapport, 9, 27, 115
Read, J. P., 136, 166
Reed, E, 164
Referrals to counseling centers for anxiety and stress, 82–84

  for eating disorders, 116–118
  for grief, 188–190
  for interpersonal violence, 155–156
  for sexual assault and victimization, 135–137
  skills of faculty and staff, 4–5, 38–41
  for substance use, 173–176
Reflecting feeling, 14, 36
Relationship development with students, 27–28, 37. *See also* Rapport
Resiliency, 49–51
Resistance to change, 36–37
Resources
  for anxiety, 197–199
  for boundaries and confidentiality, 199
  for depression, 199–201
  for eating disorders, 202–203
  for grief and loss, 204
  information giving and, 20–21
  for interpersonal violence, 204–207
  for mental health, 197–212
  psychological, 76–77
  for sexual assault and victimization, 208–210
  for stress, 197–199
  for substance use, 210–212
  for suicide and suicidal ideation, 199–201
Ritalin, 168–169
Robertson, I., 49
Rogers, A., 75, 79
Rogers, Carl, 8, 11, 14
Romantic relationships, 77. *See also* Interpersonal violence
Rosay, A. B., 150

S

Sadness, 88–91, 90*t*. *See also* Grief and loss
SAMHSA (Substance Abuse and Mental Health Services Administration), 99, 165
Schaufeli, W. B., 48
Scholarships, 163
Schueller, S. M., 46
Security, 30–31, 155
Sedatives. *See* Substance use and abuse
Self-advocacy, 65, 68
Self-care, 43–57
  burnout and, 46–49
  higher education work and, 44–45
  personal wellness and, 51–54, 55*t*
  resiliency and, 49–51
  stress and, 45–46
Self-confidence, 49–50
Self-disclosure, 3, 18–19
Self-injury, 87. *See also* Suicide and suicidal ideation
Sexual assault and victimization, 123–141
  approaching students on, 130–135, 134*t*
  case studies on, 126–128
  referrals to counseling for, 135–137
  resources for, 208–210
  signs and symptoms of, 124–130
  substance use and, 127–128, 134–135, 166
Sexually transmitted infections (STIs), 136–137, 166
Sexual orientation. *See* LGBTQIA+ students
Sexual Victimization of College Women study, 125
Shame, 114–115, 128
Sharma, K., 80

Index

Shorey, R. C., 150
Simple acceptance (Rogers), 11
Sleep issues, 82, 90, 92, 186
Smithey, M., 146
Smith-Marek, E. N., 148
Snyder, J., 148
Social anxiety, 74, 84
Social contact. *See also* Isolation and loneliness
   Greek-letter organizations and, 105–106
   parties and, 160
   resilience and, 50
   stress reduction and, 46
   suicide risk reduction and, 94–95
   wellness and, 53
Social media
   eating disorders and, 116
   popular college culture and, 160
   raising awareness of sexual assault through, 124
   stalking and, 149
   stress and anxiety from, 77
Social skills, 80
Sororities. *See* Greek-letter organizations
Soto-Marquez, J., 125
Spiritual wellness, 52, 53
Sprung, J. M., 75, 79
Stages of change. *See* Change and change model
Stages of grief and loss. *See* Grief and loss
Stalking, 149–150
"The Starfish Story" (Eisely), 196
Starting meetings, 15
Stereotypes, 62
Stice, E., 105
Stigma
   of counseling, 39

   diversity awareness and, 66–67
   mental health issues and, 3, 4, 62–63
   sexual assault and, 135
   students with disabilities and, 64
Stimulants, 167t, 168–169
STIs (sexually transmitted infections), 136–137, 166
Stress. *See also* Anxiety; Self-care
   burnout and, 46–49
   case studies on, 72–74, 79
   causes of, 76
   counseling referrals for, 82–84
   eating disorders and, 113–114
   higher education profession and, 44–45
   overview, 75–77
   personal wellness and, 51–54, 55t
   resilience and, 50–51
   resources for, 197–199
   self-care and, 45–46
   statistics on, 75–76, 87
   substance use to deal with, 45, 76, 161
   symptoms of, 45, 71–75
   underrepresented students and, 61–62
Stress management programs, 80
Student-athletes, 106, 162–163
Student organizations, 65–66, 68, 190. *See also* Greek-letter organizations
Students with disabilities, 64–66, 84, 93
Study environments, 80
Substance Abuse and Mental Health Services Administration (SAMHSA), 99, 165
Substance-free living options, 161, 175

Substance use and abuse, 159–180
- alcohol and, 164–166
- for anxiety, 83–84
- approaching students for, 171–173
- burnout and, 49
- case studies on, 162, 165
- counseling referrals for, 173–176
- marijuana and, 160, 167–168, 167t, 170
- misuse of prescribed drugs, 160, 168–169
- multiple, 170–171
- opioids and, 167t, 169
- resources for, 210–212
- sexual assault and, 127–128, 134–135, 166
- signs and symptoms of, 160–164
- stimulants and, 168–169, 167t
- for stress, 45, 76, 161
- types of abused substances, 167–171, 167t

Suicide and suicidal ideation
- anxiety and, 82
- approaching students and, 96–98
- campus response and, 98–100
- case studies on, 89, 94
- eating disorders and, 110, 118
- grief and loss, 182
- help-seeking behavior for, 98, 195
- IS PATH WARM mnemonic for suicide risk, 91, 91f
- LGBTQIA+ students and, 63
- PTSD and, 130
- resources for, 199–201
- signs and symptoms of, 92–96
- substance use and, 169

Suicide Prevention Resource Center, 99

Summarizing and summary statements, 13, 14–15, 36

Sun, J., 77
Support groups, 175, 189
Supportive language, 38
Support system, 46, 50
Surviving and Thriving During Stress (Eustis), 81–82
Sylaska, K. M., 148
Symptoms
- of anxiety, 71–75
- of eating disorders, 103–108
- of grief, 181–185
- of interpersonal violence, 144–149, 146t
- of sexual assault and victimization, 124–130
- of stress, 45, 71–75
- of substance use, 160–164
- of suicidal ideation, 92–96

Systemic racism, 68

T

Test anxiety, 78, 80–81, 84
Tone of voice, 10, 20
Training
- on cultural awareness, 67–68
- on mental health crises, 193–194

Transfer students, 75
Trauma, 50. *See also* Grief and loss; Posttraumatic stress disorder; Sexual assault and victimization
Triggers, 18–19, 94, 106, 173
Tripathi, K., 80
Turchik, J. A., 126
12-step programs, 175

U

Unconditional positive regard, 8

Underrepresented student populations. *See* Cultural and diversity awareness
Universality of struggle, 3
U.S. Loneliness Index, 194

V

Vacation time, 54
Values, challenges to, 17–18, 173
Victim advocacy centers, 136
Victim blaming, 131–132, 134
Violence. *See also* Interpersonal violence; Sexual assault and victimization
    racial, 68
    school shootings, 2
Visually impaired students, 65
Vulnerability, 19

W

Weight management. *See* Eating disorders
Wellness, 51–54, 55t. *See also* Self-care
Werneburg, B. L., 49
White, W. E., 149
"Why" questions, 154, 172
Wind-down rituals, 49
Women. *See* Gender
Wood, Mem, 117
Woolley, S. R., 9
Work–life balance
    for faculty and staff, 53–54. *See also* Self-care
    for students, 75, 79
Workplace stress, 45

Y

YES Institute, Florida, 67

Z

Zimmerman, Matt, 113